the

Glycemic Load Diet Cookbook

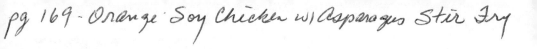

pg 169 - Orange Soy Chicken w/ Asparagus Stir Fry

the
Glycemic
Load Diet
Cookbook

150 RECIPES TO HELP YOU LOSE WEIGHT
AND REVERSE INSULIN RESISTANCE

ROB THOMPSON, M.D. & DANA CARPENDER

New York Chicago San Francisco Lisbon London Madrid Mexico City
Milan New Delhi San Juan Seoul Singapore Sydney Toronto

The **McGraw·Hill** Companies

Library of Congress Cataloging-in-Publication Data

Thompson, Rob, 1945–
    The glycemic-load diet cookbook : 150 recipes to help you lose weight and reverse
insulin resistance / Rob Thompson and Dana Carpender.
        p.   cm.
    Includes index.
    ISBN-13: 978-0-07-159739-5
    ISBN-10: 0-07-159739-5
    1. Reducing diets.   2. Glycemic index.   3. Insulin resistance.   I. Carpender,
Dana.   II. Title.

RM222.2.T4846   2009
613.2′5—dc22   2008034452

3 4 5 6 7 8 9 10 11 12 13 14 15 16 17 18 19 20 21 22 23 24 WFR/WFR 0

ISBN 978-0-07-159739-5
MHID   0-07-159739-5

McGraw-Hill books are available at special quantity discounts to use as premiums and sales
promotions or for use in corporate training programs. To contact a representative, please visit
the Contact Us pages at www.mhprofessional.com.

This book is printed on acid-free paper.

Dedicated to the memory of my father,
John Carpender. His eating habits were
disastrous, but his pride in my writing was
an endless source of joy.
—Dana

To my wife, Kathy, for her support
and encouragement
—Rob

Contents

Introduction

Welcome to *The Glycemic-Load Diet Cookbook*

Carb Science: A Note from Dr. Rob

In the past, doctors took the old saying "You are what you eat" literally. They figured you got fat from eating fat and cholesterol buildup in your arteries from eating cholesterol. In the 1960s, scientists discovered a link between high blood cholesterol levels and heart disease and made an assumption that changed the way Americans ate for decades. They assumed, without proof, that high blood cholesterol came from eating too much cholesterol. Soon government agencies began telling people to eat fewer eggs and dairy products and less red meat. Low-cholesterol diets were supposed to be not only good for your arteries but also thriftier, kinder to animals, and friendlier to the planet. How could you go wrong?

Americans actually did as they were told. Average consumption of eggs, dairy products, and red meat declined steadily for three decades. The result? People kept right on having heart attacks. Following the advice to cut cholesterol had no effect on the incidence of heart disease. Research subsequently showed that low-fat, low-cholesterol diets are ineffective for preventing heart disease and don't even lower blood cholesterol levels much.

What doctors didn't know then that they know now is that most of the cholesterol in your blood does not come from food. Your liver makes about three times more cholesterol than you eat. If you eat less, it makes more. If you eat more, it makes less. In fact, most of the cholesterol you eat passes right through your digestive tract without being absorbed at all. It's not how much cholesterol you eat that determines your blood cholesterol level; it's how readily your body gets rid of it, and that's a genetic thing. When it comes to cholesterol, who your parents are is much more important than what you eat.

Actually, there's nothing inherently wrong with reducing your fat and cholesterol intake. The problem is, if you eat less of one kind of food, you usually end up eating more of another. Sure enough, when Americans started cutting down on eggs, meat, and dairy products, they began eating more carbohydrates, but not the healthful kind—not fresh fruits and vegetables. They started eating more starch—and not just a little more but a *lot* more. By 1997, Americans were eating 48 percent more wheat, 186 percent more rice, and 131 percent more frozen potato products (read french fries) than they had in 1970.

That's a big change in eating behavior. You would expect it to have some effect. Indeed it did—a bad one. The obesity rate skyrocketed in perfect tandem with the increasing carbohydrate consumption. By 1997, the percentage of Americans who were overweight had doubled; the diabetes rate, which tracks the obesity rate, tripled.

The old mantra "You are what you eat" is misleading. Your body can quickly turn carbohydrate to fat, fat to carbs, and both to cholesterol. You definitely do not need to eat fat to get fat. Refined carbohydrates like bread, potatoes, and rice actually have more potential to make you fat than fat itself does. These foods are full of starch, and as soon as starch reaches your digestive tract, it turns to sugar. Starch delivers more sugar into your bloodstream and does it faster than any other kind of food, including sugar itself. These blood sugar surges cause your body to produce huge amounts of insulin, a hormone that, in excess, is notorious for promoting weight gain.

Starch does another peculiar thing. It short-circuits into your bloodstream in the first foot or two of your intestine. Unlike most foods, it never traverses the last twenty feet, where several appetite-suppressing hormones come from. An hour or two after you eat it, you're hungry again.

Knowing what food scientists know now about carbohydrate metabolism, it's not surprising that America's shift away from fat and cholesterol toward a diet high in refined carbohydrates caused an epidemic of obesity and diabetes.

About the time scientists were discovering a relationship between high blood cholesterol and heart disease, Dr. Robert C. Atkins, an experienced New York cardiologist, noticed that many of his overweight patients lost weight if they strictly avoided carbohydrates even as they continued to eat satisfying amounts of rich food, including plenty of fat and cholesterol. He developed a diet that restricted all carbohydrates, including sugar, grains, potatoes, and sugar-containing fruits and vegetables, but allowed dieters to eat all of the cholesterol- and fat-containing food they wanted—meat, cheese, butter, eggs, nuts, avocados, olives, and oils. His experience convinced him that low-carbohydrate, liberalized-fat diets did not cause heart disease or high cholesterol.

His timing couldn't have been worse. Government agencies had begun sounding the alarm about cholesterol, and Atkins's advice to eliminate carbs and not worry about cholesterol was anathema to them. As cholesterol fears gripped the American public, his diet fell from popularity. It took thirty years for researchers to figure out that Atkins was right. When they finally put the low-carbohydrate diet to the test, they found that subjects who eliminated carbohydrates but continued to eat unrestricted amounts of fat and cholesterol lost more weight *without even trying to cut calories* than those on low-fat diets *who tried to reduce calories*. There were no heart problems. The balance between good and bad cholesterol—the best predictor of heart disease risk—actually improved.

I have seen many patients who have tried the Atkins diet, and the results are sometimes astonishing. For some it is as if they stop ingesting a toxin that has been poisoning them for years. Fat seems to virtually melt away even as they eat plenty of rich food. Their cholesterol and blood sugar levels usually look better than ever.

You would think that a diet that allows unlimited amounts of rich food and yielded such gratifying results would be easy to follow. The problem is *food cravings*. Eliminating carbs at first might seem easy, but soon you start craving the foods that are missing. You long for more fruit, vegetables, starches, and sweets.

The result is that most people who try Atkins's radical low-carb diet give it up. The diet fell from popularity, not because of cholesterol problems—it was proved safe—and not even because of hunger since you could eat all you wanted. Irresistible cravings for the foods that were missing made the diet difficult to stick with.

These days, scientists know a lot more about carbohydrate metabolism than they did when Atkins first publicized his diet. A breakthrough occurred when researchers at the University of Toronto discovered that when it comes to their effects on blood sugar and insulin levels, not all carbohydrates are the same. Some raise blood sugar levels more than others do, despite similar carbohydrate contents. These scientists developed a way of measuring the effects of various foods on blood sugar and insulin levels called the *glycemic index*. This concept, which was only in its infancy when the low-carb movement began, evolved into a powerful tool called the *glycemic load*.

Being able to know the glycemic load of various foods is great news for people trying to avoid blood sugar surges. It narrows the list of culprits down to two kinds of foods: *starch-containing solids and sugar-containing liquids*. There is no need to worry about fruits and vegetables or even some sweets. It makes little difference whether the carbohydrate content of one is greater than another. Their glycemic loads are minor compared to those of the two main offenders, starches and sugar-containing soft drinks. Coupled with what scientists now know about fat and cholesterol, the glycemic-load measurements open the door to a style of eating that is more rich and flavorful than the way most people eat *when they aren't worrying about what they're eating*. Indeed, it's an eating style—so simple that it's hard to think of it as a diet—that's easy enough to follow for life.

Recently, the editors at McGraw-Hill and I marveled at how the glycemic load paves the way to an especially rich and flavorful, yet healthful, cuisine. We became excited about the idea of publishing a cookbook based on new concepts about diet and decided to ask the diva of low-carb cuisine herself, Dana Carpender, if she would apply her considerable talents to the task.

Dana is a nationally recognized nutritional expert and cookbook author who has published several bestselling cookbooks, including *500 Low-Carb Recipes* and *The Every Calorie Counts*

Cookbook. For years she had a nationwide syndicated column on low-carb cuisine. For years she published the e-mail newsletter *Lowcarbezine!* and has recently begun blogging at holdthetoast .com. I have been impressed with Dana's extensive knowledge of food preparation and nutrition as well as her fine food sense. Dana understands how new knowledge about nutrition can set food lovers free. All you need to do is glance at a few of her recipes to see how pleasurable reducing your glycemic load can be.

Low-Carb Cooking: A Note from Dana

The best part of my job is that people send me free stuff.

No, that's not true. The best part of my job is that I get e-mail from readers, telling me my books have changed their lives for the better. The other best part of my job is that I get to stay home with my dogs, putter around the kitchen, try new recipes, and make a living doing it.

But the best perk of my job is that people send me free stuff. Food, wine, books. Especially books. Piles and piles of books! Mostly cookbooks, which is great, because I collect them. But they send me nutrition books too.

That's how I wound up reading *The Glycemic-Load Diet* by Dr. Rob Thompson: His publisher sent me an advance copy, hoping I'd review it in print. It took me a while to get around to reading it. Then my Internet service went dead for a week, and I read three books before it came back up. One of them was *The Glycemic-Load Diet.*

I've read a lot of low-carb books, many of them very useful. I've known for a long time that different people, with their differing bodies and lifestyles and goals, find different approaches to carbohydrate restriction to be the right fit. I've never backed one form of carbohydrate restriction to the exclusion of other approaches. Communication with other low-carbers made it clear from the beginning of my journey that carbohydrate tolerance varies widely, as do people's lives and "food demons." As a result, different approaches work well for different people.

The bottom line in choosing a nutrition plan is "Can you do it forever?" Because that's what it takes, not just to keep the weight off, but to keep your blood sugar and insulin levels down and to prevent the vast and frightening array of health problems that come from high insulin and blood sugar.

The thing that struck me about Dr. Rob's *Glycemic-Load Diet* was how simple and straightforward it is. There are just two simple rules: no starches, no sugary beverages. In a field where the waters can easily be muddied by needless complexity, that's a real strength. The diet also struck me as easy to live with since it requires no counting or measuring or keeping track of anything.

I also liked that Dr. Rob's main focus is not so much weight loss as overall health, particularly helping the rapidly growing diabetic and prediabetic population avoid the nasty consequences of out-of-control blood sugar and insulin levels.

In short, I thought Dr. Rob's approach would make a lot of sense for a lot of people, and I said so, both in my column and on my website. I was instantly enthusiastic when McGraw-Hill asked me if I'd be interested in writing the companion cookbook.

I don't have any problem eating a low-carbohydrate diet. I don't struggle with it. I'm not plagued by cravings. I don't gaze wistfully at the pasta selections on menus when I go out to eat. I don't hear doughnuts calling to me. I'm a feel-good junkie. Eating this way makes me feel great, so it's what I want to do. It's that simple.

I realize this makes me something of a freak. Many people would quite literally rather die than change their eating habits—indeed, they do it every day. I hope you're not one of them. Throughout the recipes on the following pages, I'll be guiding you through the ins and outs of cooking and eating according to Dr. Rob's glycemic-load diet, drawing on Dr. Rob's expertise of course. The purpose of this cookbook is to help you slash your glycemic load and make this a permanent lifestyle change by giving you many, many answers to the pressing question "What the heck do I eat now?"

When you find the answer to that question, you will discover yourself losing weight and feeling great too. You'll wonder what took you so long.

the

Glycemic Load Diet Cookbook

1

How the Glycemic-Load
Diet Works

Before we get started, it will be helpful for you to know two definitions:

Glycemia: the presence of the sugar glucose in the blood

Glycemic: having to do with glucose in the blood

Unless you've been living under a rock, you've heard the term *glycemic* lately. A high-glycemic-load diet—a diet that raises blood sugar levels—is turning out to be correlated with most of the diseases we used to blame on fat intake: obesity, heart disease, female infertility, high blood fats, acne, insulin resistance and diabetes, even some cancers.

But what does it *mean*? What is the *low*-glycemic-load diet?

A low-glycemic-load diet (what I call simply the *glycemic-load diet* in this book for the sake of brevity) is an eating style that greatly lessens the amount of insulin your body has to make. It does this by preventing large amounts of glucose from rushing into your bloodstream all at once. Eliminating these "glucose shocks" not only helps you lose weight while continuing to enjoy satisfying amounts of good food but also can dramatically improve the way you feel and actually lengthen your life.

Before I explain this way of eating, let me give you a little background. Chances are you feel guilty about being overweight. You've been told all your life that it's just a matter of willpower, that it's all about "calories in, calories out," that all you have to do is eat less and exercise more and you'll lose weight and improve your health. If you're overweight, you *must* lack self-control. But is this true? Study after study has demonstrated that overweight people are no less disciplined than normal-weight people. No one can just dial down the number of calories he or she eats at will. We all know what the failure rate is for calorie-restricted diets. Chances are you've contributed to that statistic yourself.

Obesity results not from lack of willpower but from an imbalance in the body's hormones, substances that govern body chemistry. The best way to lose weight is to correct the underlying hormonal disturbances that caused you to gain weight in the first place. When people do that, they are often amazed at how easy it is to lose weight and keep it off. What went wrong to make you gain weight? It has to do with the way your body balances the energy you put into it versus the energy it expends.

How Your Body Uses Energy

What exactly is a calorie, anyway? A calorie is a measurement of energy. Just as we buy gasoline for our cars in gallons (or, outside the United States, in liters), we buy fuel for our bodies in calories. There are four sources of calories: protein, carbohydrate, fat, and alcohol. You may be surprised to hear that, despite all the low-fat propaganda, the biggest source of calories in the American diet by far is not fat but carbohydrate.

The main purpose of body fat is the same as the gas tank on your car: to let you carry a supply of fuel around with you to provide a steady source of energy between refuelings—in this case, between meals.

The idea behind fat-restricted diets was the belief that we literally "are what we eat"— that we get fat because we eat too much fat. If we cut dietary fat, we'd automatically eat fewer calories, and as a result we'd burn our own fat—the "fuel in the tank"—instead. The only problem is it didn't work. Twenty years of cutting fat have left Americans fatter, sicker, and more tired, not to mention with a spanking-fresh epidemic of type 2 diabetes. Why?

It turns out that there are several problems with the notion that a calorie is a calorie is a calorie: for one, we're not cars; we're complex living organisms. Unlike a car, which will run at the same rate right up to the moment when it sputters and dies for lack of fuel, your body has powerful mechanisms to balance the energy you take in with the energy you burn up. When you eat fewer calories, your body slows down. This is why low-calorie diets can make you tired—your body is trying to balance the fact that you're giving it less fuel by burning less fuel. Studies show that it is very possible for dieters' bodies to slow down so much that they won't lose weight—may even gain it—at 1,500 calories per day, which is clinically considered a semistarvation diet. The most discouraging thing about this diet-induced metabolic slowdown is that it doesn't just go away when you stop dieting. It persists for months. As a result, you actually gain weight eating fewer calories than you did before. That's right. Strict low-calories diets can actually make you gain weight.

A Tale of Two Fuels

Another difference between your body and a car is that your body is a dual-fuel machine. Your car can run on only one fuel, gasoline. But your body can run on two fuels: glucose ("blood sugar") and fat. Think about it. You've heard that you need carbohydrates for energy. You've also been told that this or that exercise will get you into your "fat-burning zone." The truth is, your body is happy to burn either fuel.

Again, the old saying "You are what you eat" is misleading. Your body can quickly turn carbs to fat and fat and protein to carbs. You don't need to eat fat to get fat, and you don't need to load up on carbs to keep your blood sugar up.

Here's the part you didn't know: *your body has to get rid of glucose before it starts burning fat.* All carbohydrates turn to glucose. If you give your body a serving of carbohydrates every few hours, your body doesn't bother to shift over to burning fat. If you have, say, cereal and juice for breakfast, a granola bar midmorning, a sandwich with a soda for lunch, pasta or a potato with dinner, and some chips in front of the television in the evening, your body can go through the whole day burning glucose instead of fat. If you have any glucose left over, your body will quickly turn it to fat and stash it on your belly, butt, or thighs.

So the question becomes "How can I get my body to burn fat instead of glucose?" The answer is simple and logical: stop giving your body all that glucose.

The Problem with Quick Energy

Maybe you have heard that carbohydrates give you "quick energy." It sounds good. But is it?

Gasoline is quick energy, so quick that if you checked your gas tank by match light you'd be lucky to survive the experience. That's why your car has fuel injectors—to turn quick energy into slow, constant energy, to feed just a tiny bit of that gasoline into the engine at a time. But your body doesn't have fuel injectors. It has no way to use carbohydrates gradually. High-carbohydrate meals simply didn't exist until mankind started farming grains and beans ten thousand years ago. That sounds like a long time, but in biological terms it really isn't. We come from hunter-gatherer ancestors who lived on meat, vegetables, and fruit in season, and our bodies are still made for that sort of diet, rather than for a diet based on grains and beans. Rapidly digestible, high-carbohydrate foods such as starch are a very recent addition to the human diet, and we simply don't have the mechanism to use big doses of it gradually.

When you eat a big dose of starch—say, a plate of spaghetti and a couple of slices of garlic bread—it all turns into glucose and floods into your bloodstream very quickly. Your blood sugar shoots up, and for the moment you feel satisfied. But high blood sugar is dangerous, and your body knows it. So it goes into action to get your blood sugar back down.

It's All About Insulin

How does your body get your blood sugar back down? It releases *insulin*. No doubt you've heard that insulin is that stuff that diabetics take. But what is it? What does it do?

Insulin is a hormone with a very specific task: it signals your body to take sugar out of your bloodstream, where it can cause trouble, and put it into your cells instead. It opens "doors" on the surface of your cells called *insulin receptors*. If you're using your muscles at that moment—walking, working out, whatever—your muscles will be able to burn some of that glucose. But if you're sitting at your desk, sitting in your car, sitting in front of the television, your muscle cells aren't going to be interested. So the insulin tells your body to convert the glucose into fat, opens the doors on your fat cells—and puts it in the tank for later.

Simply put, *insulin is the fat storage hormone*. So long as you have high levels of insulin in your bloodstream, your body will not only put fat *into* the tank; it will keep fat from going *out* of the tank. Insulin tells your body to store fuel, not tap into it.

The opposite occurs when your insulin levels fall. Your body gets the message that it doesn't have much glucose to run on and shifts over to burning fat for fuel instead. That's when your body starts to draw fuel *out* of the tank.

Think back for a moment to our hunter-gatherer ancestors, the ones who didn't eat grains and beans and therefore got only what little carbohydrate they found in wild vegetables and fruits, at least on a day-to-day basis. Most of the time, their bodies were running on fat from the game they ate. (Yes, much game is lean, but even in wild animals the organ meats, marrow, brain, and other internal tissues are rich in fat, and hunter-gatherers actually preferred these parts to the muscle meat.) When game was scarce, prehistoric humans could forestall starvation by eating vegetation. Although this was often largely indigestible carbohydrate such as grass, bark, roots, and unripe fruit, sometimes they found richer sources such as ripe fruit or even honey. Let's say they did get one big dose of carbohydrate—say they found a beehive and had a big party, eating all that honey. The honey would flood into their bloodstreams, their bodies would release insulin, and the glucose would be turned into fat and stored. No big deal. Because how often did they find a beehive? Soon they'd be back to eating game, their insulin levels would drop, and they'd shift right back to burning fat. In the meantime, the honey they ate would become fat, which they could use for fuel for a week or two. Simple and elegant.

The whole thing got messed up when we started to eat big doses of carbohydrate all the time. Indeed, modern humans consume hundreds of times more glucose in carbohydrates than their ancient ancestors did. By causing our bodies to constantly release insulin, we keep ourselves in fat storage mode. Our body takes all those calories and puts them into storage where we can't get at them, so we seem to be hungry all the time, even soon after we eat. Our muscles, organs, and appetite centers in our brain stay hungry, a state that has been called *internal starvation*. We eat plenty but never feel satisfied.

And It Gets Worse: Insulin Resistance and Type 2 Diabetes

For many of us, this constant oversue of our ability to turn glucose into fat for later turns really disastrous: our bodies stop responding to insulin, a condition called *insulin resistance*. Those "doors" on our cells, the insulin receptors, get harder and harder to open—think of them as having rusty hinges. It takes more and more and *more* insulin to open the doors and get the sugar out of our blood. Consequently, our insulin levels grow higher and higher, a condition called *hyperinsulinemia*. People with insulin resistance produce as much as *six times* the normal amounts of insulin, and that's the problem. Excessive insulin, whether given as medication or produced by the body, is notorious for causing weight gain. Indeed, most overweight people have insulin resistance.

These days, more people than ever have insulin resistance because we have become so sedentary. A hundred years ago, people weren't as susceptible as we are to obesity and diabetes because they were more physically active. All it takes is about thirty minutes of brisk walking to restore the body's sensitivity to insulin, but many of us don't even do that. We ride to work in a car or bus, sit at a desk all day, then come home and watch television. As we gain weight, exercise becomes more difficult, which contributes to insulin resistance as well. The less we use our muscles, the rustier the hinges on the doors get. As we slow down, our insulin resistance intensifies. However, the insulin receptors on our fat cells continue to work just fine long after the others start to fail. We can still store fat!

As insulin resistance progresses, our insulin levels rise as our bodies desperately try to open the doors on the cells and get the sugar out of our blood. Eventually, the poor overworked insulin-producing cells in the pancreas virtually burn themselves out, insulin production decreases, and we end up with high blood sugar all the time, which we call *type 2 diabetes*.

Stopping the Vicious Cycle

It's simple to stop the vicious cycle. Only two things are needed:

- Drastically lower your glycemic load.
- Do thirty minutes of moderate aerobic exercise—walking is just fine—four times a week.

That's it.

Excessive amounts of insulin keep you hungry and encourage your body to store energy as fat. Reducing glycemic load works to promote weight loss by preventing insulin from rising to unnaturally high levels. Research studies have repeatedly shown that people who reduce the glycemic load of their diet without even trying to cut calories *lose more weight than folks on low-fat diets who try to cut calories.*

If you just lower your glycemic load and oil the hinges of your muscle cells with moderate exercise, you reverse your insulin resistance and the insulin levels in your blood drop like a rock. Your body stops socking away everything you eat into fat storage and starts acting like the dual-fuel machine it is, burning fat instead of glucose for most of your needs. Because you have enough *fuel*, you stop feeling hungry every second of every day.

As your energy levels increase, you'll find that exercise is not such an unpleasant idea. Healthy bodies that have enough fuel like to move—just watch the kids at the playground if you doubt it. You can start easy. Walking is as good an exercise as any for losing weight and increasing insulin sensitivity. It takes only thirty minutes to open those doors on your cells. Or maybe you'd like to bike to the store, or putter around the garden, or even dance. The Russians have a wonderful phrase for it: *muscular joy.*

You'll be able to actually enjoy using your body again.

Glycemic Index Versus Glycemic Load

You hear the word *glycemic* all the time these days. Magazines recommend a "low glycemic diet," often suggesting that such a diet should be high in fruits, vegetables, and whole grains (the fruit and vegetables are OK, but the "whole grain" is wrongheaded, as we'll get to in a moment.) Ads for prepackaged diet club meals claim that they've used the "secret of the glycemic index" so that "carbs are no longer off limits."

The problem is that magazine and television ads are unclear as to the difference between glycemic *index* and glycemic *load.* Trust me. There's a big difference, and not understanding it can ruin your efforts to lose weight. So let's clarify the two terms.

We'll start with *glycemic index,* the older concept. This is a measure of how quickly any given carbohydrate food is absorbed into the bloodstream, which in turn governs how high blood sugar will rise as a result.

How is glycemic index determined? A group of people has their fasting blood sugar tested and recorded. They then eat a portion of the food to be tested. That portion is calculated carefully to contain fifty grams of carbohydrate *available for absorption into the bloodstream*—keep this point in mind, because we'll come back to it. The subjects' blood sugar is then tested at regular intervals to see how sharply it rises and falls. These results, which can vary from person to person, are then averaged out.

That average is then ranked against a "reference food"—usually pure sugar or white bread. The reference food is rated 100, and other foods are given a number indicating how they affect blood sugar in comparison to it. For example, using white bread as reference food, oranges have a glycemic index of 60, which means fifty grams of available carbohydrate in an orange will raise blood sugar 60 percent as much as fifty grams of available carbohydrate in white bread will. Even though the amount of glucose that ultimately enters your body is the same, when it is consumed in the form of an orange it raises your blood sugar less than when it is delivered in the form of white bread.

Glycemic-index tests have turned up some surprising results. For instance, in the 1970s a push started to get us to eat more *starches*: bread, potatoes, cereal, pasta, rice, and the like. It was believed that starches were absorbed more slowly than *sugar*—and that a starch-heavy diet would, therefore, lead to stable blood sugar levels and reduce hunger. The glycemic-index measurements proved this to be wrong.

For example, a baked potato has a glycemic index of 121, while sugar has a glycemic index of 115. This doesn't mean that sugar is a better food than potatoes, since the potatoes contain some vitamins and fiber, while the sugar is nutritionally empty. But it does mean that starches raise blood sugar just as much as pure sugar. In fact, fifty grams of carbohydrate from a baked potato actually raises blood sugar a little *more* than fifty grams of sugar will.

What Does Fifty Grams Have to Do with Reality?

Let's go back to a point mentioned earlier. Remember that the scientists who measure the glycemic index always use a portion that contains fifty grams of available carbohydrate. The problem with this is that it bears no resemblance to the amounts of food people typically eat in real life. It doesn't take into account that some foods simply have *a lot more carbohydrate per serving* than others do. Take carrots. They have a glycemic index of 68, high for a vegetable. But do you realize how many carrots you'd have to eat to get fifty grams of available carbohydrate? Carrots are full of indigestible fiber, which is a carbohydrate, but it does not get absorbed into your bloodstream. You would have to eat a pound and a half of carrots to get fifty grams of available carbohydrate. Nobody eats that many carrots! You'd be hard-pressed to eat enough carrots to move your blood sugar more than a point or two.

On the other hand, whole wheat pasta has a glycemic index of 53. That might sound better than carrots, but it takes only a cup and a half of pasta to get you to that fifty-gram mark of available carbohydrate—and most people eat more than a cup and a half. Very simply, people seldom consume enough vegetables to get excessive amounts of available carbohydrate but think nothing of consuming a couple hundred grams of carbohydrate in starches—pasta, rice, potatoes, bread, and the like. A typical serving of these starchy foods contains a lot more available carbohydrate than a carrot or two does—and therefore will have a bigger effect on your blood sugar, despite the lower glycemic index.

This means that the glycemic index is not a clear guide to how foods will affect your blood sugar.

Glycemic Load

Because the glycemic index doesn't tell us how foods affect people in real life, the concept of the *glycemic load* was developed. Instead of using the standard fifty grams of available carbohydrate as a test food, the glycemic load takes into consideration the amounts of food people typically eat. Food scientists have discovered that you can estimate the glycemic load of a food by simply multiplying its glycemic index by the number of grams of available carbohydrate in a typical serving: let's use white bread and whole wheat bread as examples.

White bread has a glycemic index of 100, and whole wheat bread has a glycemic index of 83, so you might think whole-grain bread would raise your blood sugar less than white bread, right? Wrong! A slice of white bread contains fourteen grams of available carbohydrate compared to twenty grams for a slice of whole-grain bread. In other words, there's just plain more food in whole wheat bread. If you multiply the glycemic indexes by the grams of available carbohydrate in a typical slice, you will find that the glycemic load of a serving of whole-grain bread is 19 percent higher than that of a serving of white bread. Using a slice of white bread as the reference food and giving it a glycemic load value of 100, the glycemic load of a slice of whole-grain bread is 119. Whole wheat bread not only raises your blood sugar 19 percent more than white bread does but contains more calories to boot. Make no mistake, whole wheat bread will not help you lower your blood sugar or your insulin levels.

Here's another example of how the glycemic load differs from glycemic index, which illustrates another important point. Let's talk about candy. Consider Life Savers. They have a glycemic index of 115, the same as pure sugar. However, a single Life Saver weighs just three grams. Because it is so small, its glycemic *load* is only 20. Here is a case where a serving of candy, which you have been told to avoid since you were in diapers, is easier on your blood sugar than a slice of whole wheat bread, which you have been told is good for you. This holds true for some other candies, including chocolate. A serving of two one-inch squares of chocolate has a glycemic load of 68, considerably less than a slice of bread.

Look at it this way: a pile of candy the size of a typical serving of potatoes would raise your blood sugar as much as a pile of potatoes would. The difference is, you usually don't need a pile of candy that big to satisfy your sweet tooth. The problem with candy is that some people have a hard time stopping, or they simply eat huge portions—candy bars have grown in size exponentially since my childhood! If you are a person who craves and binges on sweets, you are probably better off avoiding them altogether. However, as long as the serving size is small—about as much as you can wrap your fist around—it won't raise your blood sugar as much as a slice of bread.

The point is that the amount of available carbohydrate in a serving of food is at least as important as its glycemic index—if not more so.

So now you are prepared to understand the most important point of this book: although the glycemic indexes (not glycemic loads) of starches such as bread, potatoes, and rice are somewhat higher than for other foods, the glycemic *loads* are *several times higher*. As you can see from the table in this section, whether one fruit or vegetable has a higher glycemic load than another is largely irrelevant. None comes close to the blood-sugar wallop starch delivers. What the glycemic-load measurements tell you that's going to change your way of eating is that the starches aren't just a little worse than other foods. They're terrible!

But here's the good news. When you look closely at a list of glycemic loads of the most common foods we eat, you can see

Table 1.1 Glycemic Loads of Common Foods

Food Item	Description	Typical Serving	Glycemic Load
Pancake	5-in. diameter	2½ oz.	346
Bagel	1 medium	3⅓ oz.	340
Orange soda	12-oz. can	12 oz.	314
Macaroni	2 cups	10 oz.	301
White rice	1 cup	6½ oz.	283
Spaghetti	2 cups	10 oz.	276
White bread	2 slices, ⅜ in. thick	2¾ oz.	260
Baked potato	1 medium	5 oz.	246
Whole wheat bread	2 slices, ⅜ in. thick	2¾ oz.	234
Raisin bran	1 cup	2 oz.	227
Brown rice	1 cup	6½ oz.	222
French fries	medium serving, McDonald's	5¼ oz.	219
Coca-Cola	12-oz. can	12 oz.	218
Hamburger bun	5-in. diameter	2½ oz.	213
English muffin	1 medium	2 oz.	208
Doughnut	1 medium	2 oz.	205
Cornflakes	1 cup	1 oz.	199
Corn on the cob	1 ear	5⅓ oz.	171
Blueberry muffin	2½-in. diameter	2 oz.	169
Instant oatmeal (cooked)	1 cup	8 oz.	154
Chocolate cake	1 slice (4" × 4" × 1")	3 oz.	154
Grape-Nuts	1 cup	1 oz.	142
Cheerios	1 cup	1 oz.	142
Special K	1 cup	1 oz.	133
Tortilla, corn	1 medium	1¾ oz.	120
Orange juice	8-oz. glass	8 oz.	119
Cookie (lab standard, 30 g)	1 medium	1 oz.	114
Grapefruit juice, unsweetened	8-oz. glass	8 oz.	100
Banana	1 medium	3¼ oz.	85
All-Bran	½ cup	1 oz.	85
Tortilla, wheat	1 medium	1¾ oz.	80
Apple	1 medium	5½ oz.	78
Orange	1 medium	6 oz.	71
Pinto beans	½ cup	3 oz.	57
Pear	1 medium	6 oz.	57
Pineapple	1 slice (¾" × 3½")	3 oz.	50
Peach	1 medium	4 oz.	47
Grapes	1 cup (40 grapes)	2½ oz.	47
Kidney beans	½ cup	3 oz.	40

Food Item	Description	Typical Serving	Glycemic Load
Grapefruit	1 half	4½ oz.	32
Table sugar	1 round teaspoon	⅙ oz.	28
Milk (whole)	8-oz. glass	8 oz.	27
Peas	¼ cup	1½ oz.	16
Tomato	1 medium	5 oz.	15
Strawberries	1 cup	5½ oz.	13
Carrot (raw)	1 medium, 7½ in. long	3 oz.	11
Peanuts	¼ cup	1¼ oz.	7
Spinach	1 cup	2½ oz.	0
Pork	2 5-oz. chops	10 oz.	0
Margarine	typical serving	¼ oz.	0
Lettuce	1 cup	2½ oz.	0
Fish	8-oz. fillet	8 oz.	0
Eggs	typical serving	1½ oz.	0
Cucumber	1 cup	6 oz.	0
Chicken	1 breast	10 oz.	0
Cheese	1 slice (1″ × 1″ × 3″)	2 oz.	0
Butter	1 tablespoon	¼ oz.	0
Broccoli	½ cup	1½ oz.	0
Beef	10-oz. steak	10 oz.	0

that only four foods populate the top of the list: grain products, potatoes, rice, and soft drinks (including fruit juices). Simplifying further, the culprits are *starchy solids* and *sugary liquids*. These substances have two things in common: they both cause your blood sugar to shoot up; and Americans have been consuming increasing amounts of both as the obesity and diabetes rates have skyrocketed. If you do nothing else but eliminate these foods, the glycemic load of your diet and the amount of insulin your body has to make will be a fraction of what it was.

This table assigns one slice of white bread a glycemic load rating of 100 so that the glycemic loads of the other foods can be viewed in terms of percentages of that of a slice of white bread. You will find that some authors assign a slice of white bread a rating of 10. To convert one system to another, simply multiply or divide by 10. The glycemic loads of some of the foods in this table vary from those of international listings to better approximate American serving sizes.

Just Two Simple Rules: Avoid Starches and Sugared Beverages

This diet has just two rules:

- Avoid starches.
- Don't drink sugary beverages (and remember, fruit juice *is* a sugary beverage).

That's it. If you do these two things, you should keep your daily glycemic load in the healthy range—under 500. You don't have to worry about saturated-versus-unsaturated, trans fats, cholesterol, sodium, or calories. You don't have to count anything. You don't have to look anything up. You don't have to write anything down. You don't have to go hungry. And you can even have a little chocolate now and then.

By slashing your glycemic load, you'll quickly find you can trust your appetite. If you simply eat to satisfy your hunger, stop when you're full, and eat again when your hunger returns, calories will take care of themselves. By lowering your insulin levels you'll very likely find that your blood pressure, cholesterol balance, and triglycerides improve rapidly—studies show that a low-glycemic-load diet improves heart disease risk factors more effectively than fat and cholesterol restriction did.

As for trans fats, the vast majority of trans fats in your diet are coming from starchy foods, everything from crackers to microwave popcorn to commercially deep-fried foods. By cutting out the starches, you'll knock out most of the trans fats too.

Starches Versus Everything Else

To lower your glycemic load, you need to avoid foods that have a lot of carbohydrate in a serving and release it into the bloodstream fast. So which foods pack the biggest dose of carbohydrates into a serving and deliver it into the bloodstream the fastest? The answer is *starches*. If you can't forgo starches altogether, a good rule of thumb is never to eat more than a quarter serving of flour products, potatoes, or rice at any time.

What are starches? Most of the American diet. Take a look:

Bread
Rolls
Buns
Biscuits
Tortillas
Chips
Pretzels
Popcorn
Rice
All grains
Pasta, noodles, macaroni, spaghetti
Potatoes and sweet potatoes
Cereal
Cornmeal
Grits
Anything made with flour—even whole-grain flour

This is not an exhaustive list, but you get the picture.

I can feel you panicking now. "That's everything I eat!" I know. That's the problem.

What Is Starch?

Starch is a white powdery substance found in large concentrations in the seeds of plants. Each starch molecule consists of hundreds of sugar molecules linked by bonds that can be broken quickly by plant or animal digestive enzymes. The seeds of certain grasses indigenous to regions with hot, dry summers are especially rich in starch. These include wheat, barley, rice, and corn. The high concentrations of starch in these seeds provide a readily available source of sugar to jump-start seeds into sprouts during short growing seasons. No other food with the exception of pure sugar packs as many carbohydrates into as small a space as starch does.

What is it about starch that makes people gain weight? As soon as it hits your stomach, your digestive juices break it down to glucose. Starch delivers more glucose molecules into your bloodstream, and does it faster, than any other kind of food, with the exception of pure, refined sugar. Your body's insulin-producing cells have to make huge amounts of insulin to handle it, and that's the problem. Whereas small amounts of insulin actually curb appetite, excessive amounts, whether produced by your body or taken as medication, are notorious for causing weight gain.

Take a deep breath. You're going to be able to eat plenty of wonderful, flavorful, satisfying food. In fact, the food you're going to be enjoying will have far more flavor than the starches you're used to. Why? Because starch itself has no flavor. None at all.

Sugar You Can Taste Versus Sugar You Can't. Mother Nature gave us taste buds to enjoy the food we eat, including reasonable amounts of sugar, but *we have no taste buds for starch*. Except for about 2 percent of it that breaks down to sugar in our mouths, starch is tasteless. Only when it arrives in your intestinal tract does it turn to sugar. Even though starch supplies most of the calories in flour products, potatoes, and rice, whatever flavor these foods have comes from other ingredients.

What's the harm in not tasting the sugar that goes into your bloodstream? *Sugar you don't taste is more likely to make you fat than sugar you do taste.* Researchers found that sugar infused into tubes inserted into people's stomachs suppressed appetite less than sugar taken orally. If you are going to consume sugar, you're better off tasting it than letting it sneak into your stomach undetected by your taste buds.

Doubt that starch has no flavor? Try this: Put a pinch of cornstarch or white flour on your tongue. How much flavor does it have? How appealing is plain macaroni, boiled with no salt? That's starch. It's the stuff you put on it that makes it taste good—and you can have the stuff that tastes good.

Liquid Candy

The quantity of sugar-water Americans swill down has increased frighteningly over the past few decades. Somewhere along the line the standard serving went from a twelve-ounce can to a twenty-ounce bottle, a 66 percent increase. Fountain drinks are nearly big enough to swim in. Forty-two-ounce servings—far more than a quart—are not uncommon. Many people never drink anything that isn't sweetened. The black coffee of an earlier generation has turned into the mochaccino of the modern coffee kiosk. We even have a whole new class of alcoholic beverages, the sugary "alco-pops"—coolers, hard lemonades, and the like—to appeal to young adults who can't imagine drinking anything that isn't sweet.

So it is not surprising that far and away the single biggest source of sugar in the American diet is beverages. How much sugar do we get from them? That twenty-ounce bottle of cola contains fourteen teaspoons of sugar. That's more than a quarter of a cup.

Is juice better? No. Remember, you're taking the sugar out of five or six pieces of fruit and putting it in a glass. Fruit—in its natural form—is healthy. You have to bite it, chew it, and swallow it, all of which slows you down. The sweetness has time to register in your brain. The high fiber content fills you up and slows the absorption of the sugar into your bloodstream. The vitamins and minerals in it prevent food cravings. Remove the fiber—which is what juicing does—and concentrate the sugar from several pieces of fruit into one serving, and suddenly you can consume more sugar, more quickly, without feeling satisfied. How much sugar? Apple juice contains more sugar, ounce for ounce, than soda does. (Twenty ounces of apple juice contain a third of a cup of sugar!)

"But it's natural sugar!" I hear you cry. *Your body doesn't care.* Sugar is sugar is sugar. It still will raise your blood sugar.

Worse, it appears the body doesn't register sugar when we drink it rather than eat it. Scientists have discovered that unlike the sugar in solids such as candy, the sugar in liquids does not reduce the amount of other foods we eat. We just add that sugar to what we would have eaten anyway.

The only other group of foods that have glycemic loads as high as those of starches are sugar-containing soft drinks. Just one sugar-sweetened beverage a day will *double* your risk of diabetes and obesity. This includes fruit juices—orange and apple juice—as well as sodas.

Hence your second rule: *no sugary beverages*. This means no:

Sugar-sweetened soda
Gatorade and other sports drinks
Sweet tea, raspberry iced tea, and other sweet versions of
    fountain iced tea
Bottled sweetened iced tea, unless the label says *sugar-free*
Lemonade, unless the label says *sugar-free*
"Fitness waters" unless the label says *sugar-free*
"Vitamin waters" unless the label says *sugar-free*
Milk shakes
Chai
Chocolate milk and other sweetened milks
Red Bull and other "energy drinks"
Sweet coffee drinks, both bottled and from the coffee stand
Fruit juice, juice drinks, juice blends, iced tea with juice

In short, if a beverage tastes sweet, but is not artificially sweetened, it's out. If it leaves your glass sticky, it's out.

Is Natural Sugar Healthier than Artificial Sweeteners?

I'd like to tackle a question I hear a lot: "Aren't artificial sweeteners dangerous? At least sugar is natural!"

Yes, sugar is natural (although the high-fructose corn syrup that sweetens most beverages is very definitely a man-made product). So what? Tobacco is natural. Cocaine is natural. Poisonous mushrooms are natural. "Natural" does not mean "safe."

There is nothing natural about consuming the vast quantities of sugar that Americans get in beverages. There is no precedent for it that we know of in all of human history. Our bodies are not made to deal with it, *and it is killing us.*

I don't know if artificial sweeteners are 100 percent safe, but then I don't know of anything that is 100 percent safe. I am, however, convinced that they are safer than what they replace. It is best that you learn to drink far fewer sweet beverages, even diet soda—there's no evidence that diet soda has made a dent in obesity rates.

But if artificial sweeteners are what it takes to get you to stop mainlining sugar, I think they're worth it, especially as a stepping-stone to learning that a liquid need not be sweet.

So What Can I Eat and Drink?

The simple answer is *any solid that's not starchy and any liquid that isn't sweetened with sugar.* That will include:

Meat, including beef, pork, lamb
Poultry, including chicken, turkey, duck, Cornish game hen
Fish and seafood
Eggs
Cheese and other dairy products
Nuts
Seeds
Vegetables
Fruits
Fats
Coffee, hot or iced
Tea—regular and herbal, hot or iced
Artificially sweetened beverages, if you must
Sparkling water and club soda
Milk
Light beer
Wine
Spirits
And of course, good old water

In the following chapters, Dana will give you a ton of ideas for turning these foods into a rich, delicious, varied, and satisfying cuisine!

2

Going Low Glycemic Load

Before we get to the recipes, here is a variety of information that will make shifting over to a low-glycemic-load lifestyle easier for you.

Convenience Foods

Chances are you're not a "foodie." Up until you realized your health depended on changing your eating habits, you've probably depended on the same packaged, processed convenience foods that everyone else eats. You know, don't you, that you can't rely on all this starchy garbage anymore?

"But," you protest, "I have a job! I have kids! I have a million things to do! I don't always have time to cook!" Or maybe you simply hate to cook and have picked up this book out of desperation over your health issues.

Good news: there are convenience foods that fit the glycemic-load diet. Your menu will be more interesting if you cook, but you don't *have* to.

These convenience foods may put a ding in your budget. Unlike the convenience foods you're used to, these aren't based on cheap starch. But you know what? Food that makes you fat, sick, tired, and hungry wouldn't be cheap if they were giving it away.

Here are some great convenience foods that work for the glycemic-load diet:

In the Deli

- **Rotisserie chicken.** The ultimate low-glycemic-load convenience food. A rotisseried chicken plus bagged salad makes a quick and satisfying supper.
- **Deli meats.** Great for low-carb tortilla wraps, of course, but also try unsandwiches—spread your condiments between a couple of slices of cold cuts and roll them up inside a lettuce leaf, along with a slice of tomato if you like.
- **Deli salads and vegetables.** Skip the potato and macaroni salads. Look for coleslaw, roasted vegetables, sautéed green beans in olive oil, and other interesting vegetable dishes. And don't forget chicken salad and tuna salad.

In the Freezer Case

- **Frozen hot wings.** Nuke and eat. Watch out for breading.
- **Frozen hamburger patties.** Read the label to avoid starchy fillers.
- **Frozen grilled fish fillets.** These come with garlic butter, Cajun seasoning, lemon pepper, Italian herbs, and other seasonings.
- **Frozen vegetables.** I know fresh vegetables are the choice of gourmets everywhere, but I'm in favor of anything that gets you and your family to eat your darned vegetables. Just microwave, butter, and eat. Great for soups and stews too. And with a bag of stir-fry blend and some boneless, skinless chicken in the freezer, plus a bottle of your favorite stir-fry sauce on the shelf, you're never more than ten minutes away from a great meal. Be careful, though. More and more frozen vegetable blends include noodles and other starchy ingredients. Be clear on what you're getting.

- **Frozen fruit.** Frozen fruit of every kind is great to keep on hand for smoothies or for tossing into yogurt. In the winter, the frozen ones are often better than the fresh ones anyway. Use frozen unsweetened peach slices in any recipe that calls for cooking the peaches. It's a lot easier than peeling and slicing all those peaches!

In the Meat and Fish Department

- **Preskewered kabobs.** Just throw them on the grill or under the broiler.
- **Precooked ham and turkey ham.** The kind in a big oval chunk. Brown a slice or two in butter to eat with eggs or cut cubes to scramble into them. Brown a slice of ham per customer in butter, flip, and while the other side is browning, spread the top with mustard and cover with Swiss or cheddar cheese. Or just cut off a slice and stuff it in your face.
- **Cooked chicken breast strips.** Great for tossing in a salad, filling an omelet, or making a wrap sandwich in a low-carb tortilla.
- **Precooked shrimp.** Toss into a salad or dip in cocktail sauce.
- **Precooked crab legs.** Dip in cocktail sauce or go for the lemon butter.
- **Precooked bacon.** I haven't tried this, but I know people who swear by it. The best part, they say, is that you don't have all that grease to deal with.

In the Canned-Meat Aisle

- **Canned or pouch-pack tuna.** Tuna salad takes five minutes to throw together. Bagged salad tossed with bottled dressing and topped with tuna is even quicker. Tuna now comes in various flavors, by the way, but read the labels and watch out for starchy additives.
- **Canned crab, chicken, chunk ham, salmon.** See tuna.
- **Smoked salmon.** Put it in an omelet or serve it on a salad.

In the Dairy Case

- **Eggs.** It's hard to think of a way to cook eggs that takes more than twenty minutes. In particular, if you like hard-boiled eggs, keep some in the fridge at all times, ready to grab.
- **Individually wrapped cheese sticks and chunks.** These make a terrific grab-and-go breakfast or emergency rations in your purse or attaché case, though you wouldn't want to keep them in there longer than a day, of course.
- **Cottage cheese in single-serving containers with peel-off lids.** Throw one in your purse with a plastic spoon and there's breakfast. Or lunch for that matter.
- **Sugar-free yogurt in tons of flavors.** Sugary yogurt is too close to sugared beverages to be a good idea. But artificially sweetened yogurt now comes in a wide variety of flavors, and it couldn't be easier to grab and eat.

In the Produce Department

- **Precut carrots, celery, broccoli, cauliflower.** You know, all the stuff you find on a relish tray. A plate of these plus some ranch dip makes a salad or cooked vegetable unnecessary. It's a great idea to set this out as soon as you get home, for the whole family to snack on. Beats letting them fill up on chips. Grab some **grape or cherry tomatoes** while you're at it.
- **Bagged salad.** The greatest development in packaged foods in the last fifty years. Buy it. Eat it. And don't forget to try a new blend now and then.
- **Precut fruit.** Chunks of melon and pineapple, even mango. Good for snacking or fruit salad. Stash 'em in the freezer for a chilly summer treat or to throw into smoothies.
- **Salad bar.** You can make salad at the grocery store salad bar, of course. But it's also a great source of preprepped vegetables for stir-fries and other uses.
- **Guacamole.** You may be walking past the guacamole because you don't know how to eat it without chips. Stuff

it into a tomato for a killer salad! Use it to top a steak or grilled chicken breast. Combine it with Monterey Jack for the world's yummiest omelet filling.

- **Prechopped onions.** My grocery store carries diced fresh onions in plastic tubs. These can streamline everything from chili to stir-fries to slow-cooker meals.
- **Presliced mushrooms.** Sliced fresh mushrooms cost the same as unsliced. Why do the work?
- **Prechopped "stoplight" peppers.** Mixed diced red, green, and yellow peppers in plastic tubs. Throw 'em in a salad, use 'em in a stir-fry—whatever you might want chopped peppers for.

Planned Leftovers

It's a great idea to deliberately cook more than you'll eat in one meal, planning on leftovers later in the week. My sister, who is a teacher and about the busiest person I know, does this. Every weekend she'll make a big pot of soup or chili and a roast or meat loaf. Those two things, plus bagged salad or frozen vegetables, make up most of her dinners for the coming week.

In Praise of Simple Meals

You might think that a cookbook author turns out "interesting" meals every day of the week. You'd be wrong. My husband and I eat a lot of simple meals: steaks, chops, burgers (without buns, of course), roasted chicken, omelets, with a simple salad or microwave-steamed vegetable on the side for dinner; fried or scrambled eggs for breakfast. We *like* these simple meals. And we get busy too, you know.

If you're short on time, dislike cooking, or both, please do not feel obligated to cook complex dishes. Feel free to live on plain and simple cooking—in fact, you'll find a number of plain and simple recipes on the following pages to try. Go ahead and eat the same thing three days in a row. So long as you keep your glycemic load low, you'll be fine.

Eating Out

Keeping your glycemic load low while eating out is easy. I've shunned bread, rice, potatoes, and pasta for thirteen years now, and I have rarely found a restaurant where I couldn't order a meal that fit my dietary needs and tasted great too.

Four notes, the first of which is the most important:

- **Ask for what you want.** Restaurants are in a service industry; reasonable requests should be met cheerfully. It's a rare restaurant that won't substitute an extra serving of vegetables or side salad for the rice or potato. If a restaurant will not accommodate reasonable special orders, take your business elsewhere.
- **Ask questions!** If you're not sure whether a dish is appropriate, ask what's in it. Is it breaded? Is it battered? Is the soup thickened with flour or cornstarch? A good waiter will know or offer to find out. Fast-food restaurants usually have a chart of ingredients and nutritional values somewhere; ask.
- **Have the waiter take the bread basket away unless the other diners object.** Why tempt yourself, especially when you're hungry? Save your appetite for the good stuff.
- **If the starch offered with your meal is very special,** a real personal favorite of yours, here's what Dr. Rob suggests: Have the waiter bring it, but leave it by the side of your plate. Eat the rest of your meal—the protein, the vegetables, the salad, all that great stuff. If you're still hungry for the starch food at the end of your meal, eat about a quarter of it. This works, of course, only if you've got what it takes to have a few bites and leave the rest. If you know that one bite will lead to devouring the whole thing, better to ask the waiter to leave it off your plate altogether.

Standard American

Your Applebee's/Ruby Tuesday/T.G.I. Friday's sort of place. They're a cinch. Get a steak, ribs, grilled chops. Watch out for breaded "crispy" chicken, but if they have grilled or roasted chicken, that's great too. These places also have a good selection of main-dish salads, which are perfect for us. Read carefully to determine if the chicken in salads is grilled or crispy—i.e., breaded and fried. Even if the menu specifies crispy chicken, restaurants should substitute grilled chicken on request.

Barbecue Joint

Hey, it's slow-smoked meat. That's for you! Ribs, chicken, beef brisket, you name it, you can eat it. If your 'cue is seasoned with dry rub, it's perfect. If it has sauce (Mmmm—barbecue sauce . . .), go easy; most barbecue sauce is very sugary. Feel free to eat the slaw and greens, but skip the fries, hush puppies, corn bread, and baked beans. Have another rib instead. Are you a pulled-pork fan? Instead of having a sandwich, pile your pulled pork on top of a big plate of slaw, an incredible combination.

Chinese

Easy! Start with spareribs, egg drop soup, or hot and sour soup instead of an egg roll, wonton, or shrimp toast. Most stir-fries are perfect for us since they consist of meat and vegetables. Skip the rice. Be wary of sweet-and-sour dishes; the meat is usually battered. Skip the moo-shu pancakes too. (If you're taking your Chinese food home, you can use low-carb tortillas in place of the moo-shu pancakes. They work nicely.)

When you have a cold, carryout egg drop or hot and sour soup can save your life!

Corner Coffee Shops and Diners

You know the kind of place—with the rotating case of desserts up front and the waitresses who call you "Hon." These places have good salads, starting with the old classic chef's salad. Often they have a "diet plate" consisting of a bunless hamburger patty and a scoop of cottage cheese, which has been on the menu since back before low-fat mania hit, when everyone knew that if you wanted to lose weight you ate protein, not starch.

Often you can get a steak, grilled pork chops, half a grilled chicken, and other good entrees. Ask for an extra salad or veggies in place of the potato. They'll probably have good slaw too. Many coffee shops and diners serve breakfast 'round the clock, and they often have an impressive selection of egg dishes. Nothing like a big omelet or steak and eggs (hold the toast and the hash browns) to fill you up!

Deli

The traditional Jewish or Italian deli can be a 50/50 proposition: You can have any kind of cold cuts they sell; you just can't have them on bread or a roll. Fortunately, most delis offer salads too. Ask for all the innards of your favorite sandwich served on a bed of lettuce. Too, delis offer great tuna or chicken salad—eat it with a fork, not as a sandwich. You will, of course, ignore the potato and macaroni salads.

One of my favorite things about Jewish delis is that instead of getting a bread basket while you wait for your meal (and admittedly, Jewish breads and rolls are wonderful), you can almost always get a dish of kosher pickles to nosh on instead. Yum.

Greek

My favorite! Try ordering all the insides of a gyros sandwich served on top of a Greek salad instead of in a pita. Terrific! Stuffed grape leaves are popular, but usually have rice in the filling; sample just one if you must. Skip the starchy hummus; have tzatziki (cucumber-yogurt dip) instead. Dip it with veggies, not pita. Feel free to devour feta and olives.

Moussaka is likely to have bread crumbs in the meat mixture and is topped with a starch-thickened sauce, so skip it. Stick to the roasted or grilled meat and poultry dishes. Greek roasted chicken is legendary, as are Greek lamb kabobs and pork souvlaki. There are likely to be excellent vegetable dishes available as well—Greek green beans, cooked in tomato sauce, are especially good.

Italian

Italian restaurants can be rough; I've been in a few where there wasn't a single meat selection that wasn't breaded. This is changing, though; many now offer grilled chicken and fish dishes. Do the best you can. If they offer the traditional chicken cacciatore—chicken stewed in tomato sauce with peppers, onions, and mushrooms—it's a fine choice.

Every Italian meal comes with at least a side of pasta, but that's easy to fix; ask for salad or steamed veggies instead. If they offer all-you-can-eat salad, hey, eat all you can! But skip the all-you-can-eat breadsticks and the garlic bread. Skip the soup as well; most Italian soups contain starchy beans or pasta or both.

Many Italian restaurants now offer excellent main-dish salads. Hot cheese dips—spinach-artichoke-mozzarella dip and the like—are currently trendy on Italian menus. With raw vegetables instead of bread for dipping, this can make a satisfying light meal.

Japanese

Sashimi is perfect; sushi has too much rice. Miso soup is fine. Teppanyaki-style grilled meat, poultry, fish, and/or vegetable dishes are ideal. Stir-fries are fine too. Skip rice, noodles, and dumplings. Avoid tempura, because of the batter.

Mexican

Like Italian restaurants, Mexican restaurants lean toward big doses of starch, starting with that basket of chips. As with the bread basket, it's best to simply ask the waiter to take the chips away.

Mexican restaurants often have good main-dish salads, but watch out for tortilla strips, beans, and corn. Fajitas are perfect; just eat them with a fork instead of in a tortilla. Grilled beef dishes like puntas de filete and carne asada are easy to find, as are grilled shrimp and chicken dishes. Mexican stews are good and usually don't contain potatoes. Carnitas—meltingly tender chunks of simmered and then browned pork—are fantastic. One of the best meals I've ever had was at a cheap joint in San Diego where they sold carnitas by the pound. I piled them on a salad, topped them with guacamole, and was in heaven.

Speaking of guacamole, it's not only delicious but great for you. Order extra and pile it on salads, fajitas, steaks—or just eat it with a fork. You should steer clear of tortillas, rice, and refried beans. This rules out tacos, burritos, enchiladas, chimichangas, and flautas. Sorry!

Pizza Parlor

Thick-crust pan pizza is out! Dr. Rob suggests that you get the thinnest-crust pizza you can find and leave the thick edge behind. Or you can order your pizza with a ton of toppings—extra cheese, pepperoni, sausage, peppers, mushrooms, anchovies, whatever you want. Then peel those toppings off the crust and scarf them down, leaving the starchy crust behind. (It helps if the pizza's had a couple of minutes to cool. Then the cheese pulls off in a solid layer, with all the other stuff attached.) The toppings are the good part, anyway. The crust is just an edible napkin.

Many pizza places have good salads, with Italian vinaigrette dressing, and lots of red onion and olives, and those pickled hot peppers. There's your side dish, if you want one.

You know that stuff like "cheesy bread," breadsticks, garlic bread, etc., is out. Pizza places love to load you up on this stuff to make it look like you're getting a great value, but that white flour cost them next to nothing—and will cost you big-time.

Seafood

If you're a seafood fan, this is one of the best possible types of restaurant for you. Any grilled, steamed, boiled, baked, or sautéed fish or seafood is likely to be fine. Just watch out for dishes that are breaded and fried, baked dishes topped with bread crumbs, and any dish where the fish is combined with pasta or rice. You'll skip the baked potato and the bread basket, of course. But feel free to dip your lobster and crab in melted butter!

Steakhouse

Can it get any better than a steakhouse for a low-load diet? Any steak you want is just fine. These places often have chicken and seafood too, but again, watch out for breading. Of course you'll skip the baked potato or fries. Ask for an extra salad or order of steamed veggies instead. And those "onion blossom" things or the more common onion rings? They're crack in food form, but they're also coated in batter. If you can't limit yourself to one or two—I know I have a hard time!—better to avoid them altogether.

Steakhouses often have salad bars. All the vegetables are fine, of course. So is any fresh fruit they may offer. Skip the croutons and Chinese noodles—if you want a little crunch, sunflower seeds or bacon bits are better choices. Pretend the pasta, potato, and bean salads aren't there.

Fast Food

Contrary to popular belief, it is possible to eat fast food and be perfectly healthy. Most fast-food places offer low-glycemic-load options—it's up to you to choose them! However, if the smell of fryer grease goes to your head, and you can't get out of a fast-food joint without eating fries or gulping a shake, you'd do better to simply stay away.

Here's a quick rundown of the low-glycemic-load options at the most popular fast-food places:

McDonald's, Burger King, Wendy's, Jack in the Box, and Arby's all offer main-dish salads. These are the obvious choice. Often you'll have the choice of grilled or crispy chicken—remember that *crispy* means "breaded"—so go for the grilled chicken. Leave off starchy toppers like croutons and Chinese noodles. You can, of course, also have a burger without the bun on top of a side salad.

Hardee's has no salads, but its West Coast version, Carl's Jr., offers a charbroiled chicken salad, perfect for us. Both Hardee's and Carl's Jr. offer particularly big hamburger patties, nice when you're leaving off the bun. You might ask for extra lettuce and tomatoes. Carl's Jr. also has a burger with sautéed portobello mushrooms, which sounds darn good to me! Hardee's and Carl's Jr. both offer chargrilled chicken sandwiches. Again, leave off the bun, ask for extra lettuce, tomatoes, and mayo, and you've got a simple but healthful meal.

If you're lucky enough to live in In-N-Out Burger territory, you can order its famous burgers "protein style"—wrapped in lettuce.

White Castle is a dead loss, not a thing for us on the menu. I've never been able to fathom the popularity of "sliders" anyway—those hamburger patties are the size of postage stamps. Go somewhere where they're more generous with the protein.

Taco Bell has only one low-glycemic-load selection: Order a taco salad, either beef or chicken. Ask them to hold the beans and double the meat. Then don't eat the taco shell! (If you can't resist the taco shell, best go elsewhere.)

Subway is a great choice. All of its sandwich fillings can be ordered as salads, with lettuce, cucumbers, peppers, and other great veggies added. Quizno's is Subway's biggest competitor. It offers five main-dish salads. Just ignore the little triangles of flatbread stuck in the sides—or if your will is weak, ask them to hold the bread. Quizno's also has a broccoli-cheese soup that should be reasonably OK for us.

Long John Silver's manages to make fish unhealthful; all its selections are breaded and fried, and with the exception of coleslaw, all the side dishes are starchy. Go somewhere else.

For a few years, KFC was my favorite fast-food place. Then it eliminated its "Tender Roast" chicken, and I was so disappointed I haven't darkened KFC's doorstep since. All the chicken at KFC is breaded and fried. I won't even talk about the god-awful "Famous Bowls," huge gloppy piles of multiple varieties of starch.

However, KFC has a couple of main-dish salads on the menu, available with either roasted or crispy chicken. Choose the roasted chicken! There are also a few side dishes at KFC that are OK—the slaw, the green beans, and the side salad—but what's the point of side dishes without a main course? I trust I don't have to tell you to stay away from the biscuits, mashed potatoes, mac-and-cheese, and so forth.

Popeyes also offers only breaded and fried chicken. Its seafood is breaded and fried as well. Some Popeyes offer a shrimp creole that should be OK if you get it without the rice, but that's about it—they don't even have main-dish salads. I'd skip it.

If you live in Boston Market territory, it's one of your best choices. You can get roasted chicken or turkey and even roast sirloin. Boston Market has salads and slaw, green beans, steamed mixed vegetables tossed in olive oil, spinach in garlic butter, and creamed spinach.

Kenny Rogers Roasters, similar to Boston Market, offers plenty of good choices—roasted chicken, of course, but also roasted turkey and barbecued ribs. (Go easy on the sugary barbecue sauce.) They have main-dish and side salads, herbed Italian green beans, creamy spinach with Parmesan, grilled vegetables, and mixed peas and carrots too.

Chick-fil-A offers a couple of chargrilled chicken salads that are fine. It also has fruit salad, coleslaw, "chicken salad cups," and side salads. Avoid the "chicken strips" salad; the chicken is breaded and fried.

What Can I Eat for Breakfast?

Dr. Rob tells me his patients have an especially hard time figuring out what to eat for breakfast, so I thought I'd give you some ideas. You've heard that breakfast is the most important meal of the day. What makes it so important?

Breakfast determines both your hunger and your energy level for the rest of the day. In one study on the effects of breakfast on hunger, the folks who ate a high-glycemic-load breakfast of instant oatmeal ate 81 percent more calories during the rest of the day than the folks who ate a cheese omelet, *even though the two breakfasts had the same number of calories.* The folks who had the omelet simply were not hungry. That, my friend, is a trick you cannot afford to miss. Breakfast is what is going to keep you away from the vending machines and the doughnuts in the break room.

So you need a high-protein, low-glycemic-load breakfast. This presents a problem if you're accustomed to eating cereal, toast, muffins, sweet rolls, or other starchy, sugary breakfasts. They will not do.

Short on time? You and the rest of the world. But breakfast is so important to your long-term success that it's worth setting your clock 10 minutes earlier. That's all it takes to scramble a couple of eggs and eat them. If you have a good nonstick skillet, all you have to do is wipe it with a paper towel and put it back on the stove, ready for the next day.

Do not hesitate to eat eggs daily. Forget everything you've heard about eggs being bad for you. They're one of the best possible foods. Enjoy 'em fried, scrambled, poached, boiled, in omelets, however you like. Lose your guilt about breakfast meats as well. Sausage and ham are good sources of protein. Bacon, not so much; have some eggs with it! You'll find pancake recipes in Chapter 4. Make them over the weekend and stash them in your refrigerator. Then warm up one or two every morning, for a quick and easy breakfast.

Don't like traditional breakfast foods? Have a hamburger patty, a chop, a steak. Warm up last night's leftovers. If you have an electric tabletop grill—you know, the George Foreman sort of thing—throw a couple of sausage patties, a hamburger, or a chop in it, set a timer for five to seven minutes, and go dress and brush your hair while it cooks.

Can't deal with hot food first thing in the day? Consider:

Cottage cheese with fruit

All-Bran, All-Bran Extra Fiber, or Fiber One cereal. These are the only cold cereals with a glycemic load low enough to fit into this way of eating. Serve with milk, or stirred into yogurt, with some fruit.

Low-carb bread toasted and spread with cottage cheese and low-sugar jam or jelly

Cinnamon, Flax, and Bran Granola (see Chapter 4)

Yogurt, either by itself or in a Yogurt Parfait (see Chapter 3)

Strawberry Smoothie (see Chapter 3)

Applesauce Spice Cake (see Chapter 12)

Nadine's Miracle Bran Muffins (see Chapter 4)

Breakfast Custard (see Chapter 3)

Lemon-Vanilla Cheesecake (see Chapter 12)
Individually wrapped cheese chunks (thrown into your purse
    or briefcase)
Hard-boiled eggs (also go in your bag)

A Few Ingredients You Should Know About

Shirataki Noodles

There is one truly low-starch noodle. Indeed, it's a low-*everything*
noodle. Let me introduce you to shirataki. Shirataki noodles are
made of virtually nothing but fiber and water. The shirataki in my
fridge claim to have 1 gram of carbohydrate, 1 gram of fiber, and
no calories at all. I call them "nothing noodles."

There are two varieties of shirataki noodles, traditional and
tofu shirataki. The traditional noodles are clear, with a jellylike
consistency and very little flavor of their own. They are distinc-
tively Asian. As a result, I find they really work only in Asian
dishes—they were truly weird with tomato sauce and Parmesan.
But they're a great choice for sesame noodles, pad Thai, Asian
noodles and broth, you name it.

Tofu shirataki are white and have a consistency that is closer
to that of wheat noodles. They, too, are quite bland. They're the
noodles to choose if you're making more traditional Western-style
dishes. I've made fettuccine Alfredo and a very good mac-and-
cheese with the tofu shirataki. They're also good in tuna-noodle
casserole.

Tofu shirataki come in two widths, spaghetti width and fettuccine width.

Both traditional and tofu shirataki come already hydrated, in a
plastic pouch full of liquid. To use them, you snip the pouch open
and pour the noodles into a strainer in your sink to drain. You will
notice that the liquid smells fishy. Panic not. Soaking the noodles
in warm water for twenty minutes or so—while you assemble the
rest of your dish—will dispel the smell. I haven't noticed the noodles actually tasting fishy.

Shirataki noodles are a lot longer than the spaghetti and fettuccine you're used to, and the traditional version resists being

bitten off! So take your kitchen shears and snip, willy-nilly, across the mass of noodles four or five times. This will take care of the problem.

Find shirataki noodles at Asian markets and some health food stores. Shirataki can be ordered from Internet retailers as well. They keep for up to a year if refrigerated, so feel free to stock up.

Guar or Xanthan

What the heck are these? Sound awful, don't they? Yet you've been eating guar and xanthan all your life. They're widely used in the food processing industry, as thickeners—which is exactly how you're going to use them.

Sauces, gravies, soups, stir-fries, and many other dishes call for flour, cornstarch, or arrowroot as thickeners. But all of those are starches, and highly refined starches at that. Guar and xanthan are, instead, finely milled, tasteless soluble fibers. They give a nice, velvety texture to gravies, soups, and sauces and add no flavor of their own.

Guar and xanthan are very similar; use them interchangeably. The easiest way to use whichever you buy is to keep it in an old saltshaker by the stove. When your sauce, soup, or gravy needs thickening, simply sprinkle the guar or xanthan lightly over the top, whisking as you do so. Stop when your dish is just a little less thick than you'd like it to be, since it will continue to thicken a little on standing.

What you should *not* do is dump a spoonful of guar or xanthan into your dish, then try to whisk it in. You'll get a big lump of jellylike stuff in the middle of your food.

Guar and xanthan are available at health food stores and online. A little goes a long way, so you shouldn't have to repurchase often. And they keep forever, so long as they don't get wet.

Vital Wheat Gluten

Gluten is a protein found in grains. When you add moisture and knead gluten, it becomes stretchy. It's that stretchy quality that allows bread dough to hold in the carbon dioxide created by growing yeast in a billion tiny bubbles, making bread rise. Rye, oats, and barley have a little gluten in them, but wheat has the most. This is why most recipes, even for rye or oatmeal bread, call for at least some wheat flour too.

But you can't use more than a little bit of wheat flour because of all that starch. The good news is you can replace much of it with fiber and protein powder. So use separated gluten, or *vital wheat gluten*, to replace the starchy regular flour.

The labeling on vital wheat gluten can be confusing. Some companies label it *vital wheat gluten*, while others just call it *wheat gluten* or *gluten*. Others call it *gluten flour*, but usually gluten flour is starchy white flour with some extra gluten added to it. How to tell? Read the label. A quarter cup of vital wheat gluten should have about forty-seven grams of protein and only about three grams of carbohydrate.

Gluten sensitivity is common; it's one of the reasons grains are not great foods for many people. I'm afraid I don't know of a substitute for gluten in my bread recipes. If you're sensitive to gluten, you'll simply have to skip them. Sorry.

Find vital wheat gluten at health food stores and sometimes in the baking aisle of big grocery stores. I use Bob's Red Mill brand.

Vanilla Whey Protein

Whey is the liquid part of milk. Protein powder made from whey is extremely nutritious, has a mild flavor, and works well for making smoothies and for replacing part of the flour in a lot of recipes. You can buy vanilla whey protein at health food stores, GNC stores, and anywhere that sells supplements for bodybuilders.

Rice Protein Powder

Rice protein powder is useful in savory dishes, where vanilla whey would taste funny. I use NutriBiotic brand, which I special-order through my health food store. If your health food store doesn't have rice protein powder, no doubt it can special-order it for you too.

Almond Meal

Almond meal is useful as a substitute for flour and cornmeal. Many grocery stores carry almond meal; check the baking aisle. However, almond meal is simple to make yourself. Just dump shelled almonds into your food processor and run it till you have a meal about the texture of coarse cornmeal.

Store almond meal in a snap-top container or resealable plastic bag in the fridge or freezer.

Pumpkin Seed Meal

Having written a slew of recipes using nut meals, I found myself getting e-mails from readers with nut allergies, wanting an alternative. I hit on pumpkin seed meal. This light-green meal works as well as almond meal in baking. It's cheaper and higher in minerals too.

I know of no commercial source of pumpkin seed meal. No big deal, though; it's a snap to make your own. Raw, shelled pumpkin seeds are available at health food stores and at Mexican markets, where they're called *pepitas*. Dump the pumpkin seeds into your food processor and run it till they're the texture of coarse cornmeal. Store in a snap-top container in the fridge or freezer.

Flaxseed Meal

Flaxseed is a true superfood. It's high in protein and fiber and one of the best plant sources of omega-3 fatty acids. It's also high in lignans, an antioxidant that may protect against estrogenic forms of cancer, like breast cancer. All this, and it has a nice, mild, nutty flavor too.

I'm not going to tell you to make your own flaxseed meal. Flax seeds are widely available, but they're tough to grind. Fortunately, flaxseed meal is now widely distributed. Health food stores carry it, and many big grocery stores have it in the baking aisle. I use Bob's Red Mill Golden Flaxseed Meal.

Store flaxseed meal in a snap-top container or resealable plastic bag in the freezer. The healthy oils in it are perishable and degrade pretty rapidly once the seeds are ground, so the freezer is preferable to the fridge unless you're likely to use it up quite quickly.

Oat Bran

This is the outside coat of the oat grain. It's high in fiber, which lowers its glycemic load. I find oat bran useful in baked goods and also as a substitute for bread crumbs or crushed cereal in meat loaves and the like. You can find oat bran in the cereal aisle with the oatmeal.

Wheat Bran

The outside coat of the wheat grain. It's loaded with insoluble fiber, which helps keep your digestive tract healthy. Available at most grocery stores and all health food stores.

Wheat Germ

Wheat germ is the little bit inside a wheat kernel that would have actually become the plant. It's the part of the wheat kernel where most of the protein and vitamins are. I've included modest quantities of wheat germ in a couple of recipes to give them a grainy flavor without much starch. I recommend raw wheat germ, since you're going to cook it anyway. Raw wheat germ is available at health food stores and sometimes in the baking aisle of grocery stores. If you can't find it, go ahead and use the toasted wheat germ you find in the cereal aisle. Store wheat germ in the fridge.

Vege-Sal

Vege-Sal is a seasoned salt, but it's nothing like traditional "seasoned salt." Instead it's salt mixed with powdered, dried vegetables. The flavor is subtle, but I think it improves many recipes. In many recipes I've given you a choice of using Vege-Sal or salt. Widely available at health food stores.

Chili Garlic Paste

Also known as *chili garlic sauce*, this Southeast Asian condiment consists largely—as you would expect—of hot chilies and garlic. Once you have it in your refrigerator, you'll find hundreds of ways to use it. Look for chili garlic paste at Asian markets or the international foods aisle of big grocery stores. So long as it's refrigerated, chili garlic paste appears to keep nearly forever.

Low-Sugar Preserves

I prefer these, not only because they have less sugar than regular preserves but also because I think they taste better. I use Smucker's brand low-sugar preserves. But if you like, use whatever you have on hand.

Bouillon Concentrate

Bouillon concentrate adds flavor to many dishes. I like Better Than Bouillon jarred paste concentrate, because unlike many bouillon granules or cubes it actually contains chicken or beef or ham or whatever flavor is listed on the label. If you can't find Better Than Bouillon, buy granules or liquid concentrate in preference to cubes, which are more difficult to dissolve.

Fish Sauce

A traditional Southeast Asian condiment, also known as *nuoc mam* or *nam pla*. Fish sauce is widely used in Thai and Vietnamese cooking. Look in the international aisle of your big grocery store or at an Asian market. Fish sauce doesn't go bad or need refrigeration.

Coconut Oil

Coconut oil has been shunned for the past few decades because it is very highly saturated. Turns out that despite—or possibly because of—that, coconut oil is very healthful stuff. It is rich in lauric acid, a fat that stimulates metabolism by improving thyroid function. Despite being saturated, lauric acid tends to lower LDL "bad" cholesterol and raise HDL "good" cholesterol. Medical studies in India, where coconut oil is a traditional cooking fat, found that when it was replaced by less saturated oils, the rates of both heart disease and type 2 diabetes *increased*. Add to this that because of being very saturated, coconut oil does not turn rancid easily. Except for extra-virgin coconut oil, which does have a pleasant coconut odor, coconut oil is quite bland. I use it often for frying and also as a substitute for trans fat–laden hydrogenated vegetable shortening. Coconut oil can be found at Asian markets and in the international aisle of big grocery stores.

Low-Carb Tortillas

These are more like flour tortillas than corn tortillas. Much of the flour is replaced with fiber and a little soy protein. I prefer La Tortilla Factory brand, because they're the highest in fiber—and therefore lowest in digestible, absorbable carbohydrate—of any low-carb tortilla I've tried. They're a staple at my house; we use them for quesadillas, wrap sandwiches, breakfast burritos, even as pizza crusts. If you can't find them in your hometown, you can order low-carb tortillas online. They keep pretty well, so order enough to last you for several weeks.

Canned Black Soybeans

Most beans are pretty starchy. They have a low-enough glycemic load that you can eat them in moderation, but large doses may spike blood sugar, especially when they're mashed or pureed. Soybeans are the exception, and black soybeans are the least starchy of the bunch. Soybeans are a pain to cook at home; they take forever to get soft. But Eden brand canned black soybeans are available at health food stores and even in the health food section of some big grocery stores. They're awfully bland on their own, but they're good in chili and some soups. If you can't find black soybeans, any canned soybeans can be substituted.

Sucanat

Sucanat is sugarcane juice that has been dried and ground into a coarse powder. It tastes a lot like brown sugar, but it's not sticky like brown sugar. It has vitamins and minerals that brown sugar lacks. You can buy Sucanat at health food stores. If you can't find it, brown sugar will work but has no vitamins or minerals.

Some of you may be wary of all concentrated sugars, this one included. I don't blame you; I feel the same way. I have used Sucanat in developing these recipes, and I haven't noticed any ill effects, but I don't use it much in my day-to-day cooking. I have too scary a history of sugar addiction.

If you prefer not to use Sucanat, you may substitute brown sugar–flavored maltitol, which is available through online specialty merchants, or brown sugar Splenda blend, which combines Splenda with brown sugar. You can also substitute Splenda plus a little blackstrap molasses, but this will change the texture of your finished product a bit.

Splenda

Splenda is the sweetener I reach for most often. I think it tastes very good, it works in a wide range of applications, it doesn't lose sweetness when heated, and because it has the same degree of sweetness as sugar, it can be substituted one-for-one, making it easy to gauge how much to use. While you are allowed some sugar on the glycemic-load diet, I am still wary of the stuff. I have often given you the choice between using a little Splenda and using a little sugar.

All measurements for Splenda in this book are based on Splenda Granular, not the Splenda that comes in the little packets. The Splenda in the packets is sweeter than Splenda Granular. If you want to substitute, you may. One packet of Splenda has the same sweetness as two teaspoons of Splenda Granular or of sugar. This means that forty-eight packets equal one cup of Splenda or sugar.

Many recipes in this book offer you a choice between using Sucanat or sugar and using Splenda. In those recipes, the first sweetener listed is the sweetener analyzed for.

3

Eggs and Dairy

O f all the nutritional slander of the low-fat era, none is so wrongheaded, so downright dangerous, as the demonizing of eggs. Please, please, do not be afraid of eggs. There is nothing more nutritious on the planet—or at your grocery store. Should you throw away the yolks? Only if you want to discard most of the vitamins, minerals, and antioxidants along with them.

It seemed intuitively obvious that eating cholesterol would cause high blood cholesterol, but the research doesn't back up the hypothesis. Even the American Heart Association has reluctantly admitted that eggs don't appear to increase heart disease risk factors. (Nor does eating high-cholesterol foods as a group.)

So eat eggs! Not just for breakfast, but anytime you want a quick, satisfying, and delicious meal. Eggs can be downright cheap, but I'd like to recommend that if they're available near you and your budget can stretch, you buy pastured eggs from small local farms. They're superior, in both flavor and nutrition.

If you can't find or afford pastured eggs, conventionally raised eggs are still a nutritional bargain. Buy them by the eighteen-egg carton. And a word to the wise: kept refrigerated, eggs will be OK

Dr. Rob Says: Are You Really What You Eat?

A lot of people, even some doctors, take the old saying "You are what you eat" literally. They think that people get fat from eating fat and get high blood cholesterol from eating cholesterol. What they don't realize is that the human body can quickly convert carbs to fat, fat to carbs, and either to cholesterol. That potato you ate? Within a couple hours, your body turns it to fat.

As for cholesterol, your liver makes about three times more than you eat. If you eat less, it just makes more. If you eat more, it just makes less. Don't blame your diet for high blood cholesterol. Blame your parents. It's mainly a genetic thing.

for omelets, casseroles, and boiling for at least six weeks. When they're a loss-leader sale item in the spring, buy as many cartons as you can fit in the refrigerator.

I'm going to assume you already know how to fry, scramble, or boil an egg and not take up space with recipes for those preparations. But they're all fine ways to cook eggs; enjoy them whenever you like.

Omelets

If I could teach everyone one cooking skill, it would be how to make an omelet. There is no other skill that allows you such a tremendous range of fast and fabulous meals. Too, when you first cut your glycemic load, it can seem odd to eat fried or scrambled eggs without toast on the side. But somehow an omelet seems like a complete meal all by itself.

Fortunately, omelets are a whole lot easier than rumor would have you believe. Here's how:

You'll need the right pan—a seven- to nine-inch skillet with a good nonstick coating and sloping sides is ideal.

Get prepared. Once you start making your omelet, things go very quickly, so have your omelet filling standing by. If you're using sautéed vegetables, sauté them first and have them standing by. If you're using cheese, grate or slice it ahead of time. If you're making an omelet to use up leftovers—a superb idea—warm them in the microwave first. Have a spatula by the stove too.

Whether you're using a nonstick skillet or cooking spray, put your not-sticky skillet over medium-high heat. While it's heating, crack two eggs into a bowl and use a fork to scramble them up. Unless the recipe says otherwise, don't add a thing—just mix up your eggs.

When your skillet is hot, add a little oil or butter. Slosh it around to cover the bottom of the skillet.

Drip one drop of the beaten eggs into the skillet. If it immediately sizzles and sets, your skillet is ready. (If the egg doesn't sizzle and set, let it heat a little more.) Dump in the beaten eggs all at once. Now comes the important part: Don't just let your eggs sit there. If you do, your eggs will be hopelessly overdone on the bottom before the top is set. An omelet is built up in layers.

So grab that spatula you set by the stove. Start lifting the edges of cooked egg and letting the still-liquid egg run underneath. Do this all around the edge, using your other hand to tilt the skillet to let the raw egg run underneath. Within a minute or so, you won't have enough liquid egg left to run.

Now turn your burner down to the lowest setting. (If you have an electric stove, it's a good idea to use two burners, the first on medium-high and a second on low, and switch burners.) Spread your filling over half of your disk of egg. Cover the skillet and let the omelet cook for a couple of minutes.

Now take a peek. If the top surface is cooked, and your cheese, if you're using any, is melted, it's done. If your omelet still looks underdone, cover it again and give it another minute or two.

When your omelet is done, slip your spatula under the naked side of your omelet and fold it over the filling. Lift the whole thing onto a plate and serve. (If you're making omelets for several people, have your oven on its lowest setting and keep the first ones warm in there as the later ones cook.)

That's it! It takes far less time to do than it's taken me to write this out. What to put in your omelet? All sorts of things. How about:

Avocado slices and Monterey Jack, topped with salsa
Sautéed mushrooms and onions
Crumbled Italian sausage, cooked with peppers and onions, topped with pasta sauce
Shredded mozzarella, topped with jarred pizza sauce
Leftover chili, plus cheddar cheese, topped with sour cream
Leftover tuna salad, plus Swiss cheese
Sliced ham and cheese, Swiss or cheddar, plus a smear of mustard
Smoked salmon and cream cheese
Raw spinach, crumbled feta, and chopped olives
Sliced turkey and tomato, plus crumbled bacon
Guacamole, tomatoes, and cheese

Almost anything that's good in a sandwich is good in an omelet, as are many dips. Once you get in the omelet habit, you'll find yourself looking at recipes thinking, "Y'know, that combination would be good in an omelet."

Here are a few recipes to get you started.

Apple, Cheddar, and Bacon Omelet

Apples and cheese are a classic combination, and so are cheese and bacon. Put all three together and—wow!

¼ apple
2 teaspoons butter
¼ teaspoon Sucanat or Splenda
2 eggs
1 ounce sharp cheddar cheese, shredded (about ¼ cup)
2 slices bacon, cooked, drained, and crumbled

Trim the core out of your apple quarter and cut into five or six slices. Melt the butter in your omelet pan and add the apple slices. Sauté over medium heat for 4 or 5 minutes, flip, and sprinkle with the Sucanat or Splenda. When the apple slices are soft and a little browned, remove from the skillet.

Give your skillet a squirt of nonstick cooking spray and put it back over medium-high heat. Beat up your eggs with a fork and make your omelet according to the omelet method at the beginning of the chapter. Put the cheese in first, then the apple slices and half the crumbled bacon. When you've folded and plated your omelet, top with the rest of the bacon and serve.

1 serving, with 406 calories, 32 g fat, 22 g protein, 7 g carbohydrate, 1 g fiber

Avocado, Bacon, and Spinach Omelets

I decided to make this recipe for two omelets because leftover avocado might turn brown in the fridge. If you want to halve this recipe, coat the cut side of your leftover avocado half with lime or lemon juice, drop it in a resealable plastic bag, seal it most of the way, then suck the air out before you finish sealing the bag. This will keep it from browning for a day or two.

> **4 eggs**
> **2 ounces Monterey Jack cheese, sliced or shredded (about ½ cup)**
> **½ cup fresh baby spinach**
> **1 avocado, pitted, peeled, and sliced**
> **2 scallions, including the crisp part of the greens, sliced**
> **4 slices bacon, cooked and drained**

Assemble all your filling ingredients by the stove.

Make your omelets one at a time, according to the directions at the beginning of this chapter. Layer each with half the cheese, then half the spinach, avocado, and scallion. Crumble two slices of bacon over that. When the omelet is folded and plated, put it in a warm spot or put a big pot lid over it while you repeat the process with the second half of the ingredients; then serve.

2 servings, each with 478 calories, 39 g fat, 24 g protein, 10 g carbohydrate, 3 g fiber

Sort-of-Indian Omelet

I adapted this recipe from the wonderful Indian cookbook *5 Spices, 50 Dishes*, by Ruta Kahate, using what I had in the house. I haven't tried the authentic version, but this version's great. As you'll see, in this omelet you just mix the fillings right into the eggs.

> 2 eggs
> 2 tablespoons minced onion
> 1 clove garlic, minced
> 1 tablespoon finely diced tomato
> 1 tablespoon minced fresh cilantro
> ⅛ teaspoon chili garlic paste
> Pinch salt
> Pinch ground turmeric
> 2 teaspoons coconut oil

Whisk the eggs; then stir in everything else but the oil.

Give your 9-inch skillet a squirt of nonstick cooking spray and put over medium-high heat. Add the coconut oil; slosh it around as it melts to coat the bottom of the skillet and let it get hot.

Add the egg mixture and let it cook, without stirring, till the edges are set. Then start the process of lifting the edges and letting raw egg run underneath, keeping in mind that with all that yumminess in the beaten egg it won't run as easily.

When there's not enough raw egg left to run underneath, carefully flip your omelet. It should be golden brown on the cooked side. Let the other side cook for a minute or so; then serve.

The book I adapted this from said that tomato ketchup was mandatory with this sort of omelet, but I think it's fine without. Do as you like.

1 serving, with 225 calories, 18 g fat, 12 g protein, 4 g carbohydrate, 1 g fiber

Spring in the Wintertime Scramble

If you're feeling too lazy to bother with an omelet, you can always just scramble wonderful tidbits into your eggs. Charmingly simple and fresh-tasting.

> ¾ cup sliced mushrooms
> 2 teaspoons minced red onion
> 2 teaspoons butter
> ¾ cup frozen peas
> 3 eggs
> Salt and pepper to taste

Give your medium skillet a shot of nonstick cooking spray and put it over medium-low heat. Start the mushrooms and onions sautéing in the butter.

Meanwhile, put the frozen peas in a small microwavable dish, add a couple of teaspoons of water, cover, and give them just a minute on high in the microwave.

When the mushrooms have changed color and softened, drain the peas and add them to the skillet. Stir 'em into the mushrooms and onions.

Now break your eggs into a dish and mix 'em up with a fork. Pour them into the skillet and scramble till set. Plate, salt and pepper, and eat!

1 serving, with 363 calories, 21 g fat, 23 g protein, 19 g carbohydrate, 6 g fiber

Savory Scramble

Bacon and eggs, only more exciting.

> 2 teaspoons butter
> 3 scallions, including the crisp greens, sliced
> 3 eggs
> 1 tablespoon half-and-half
> ¾ teaspoon brown mustard
> ⅛ teaspoon pepper
> ⅛ teaspoon salt
> 3 slices bacon, cooked and drained
> 1 tablespoon chopped fresh parsley

Give your medium skillet a shot of nonstick cooking spray and put it over medium heat. Melt the butter and throw in the scallions.

While that's happening, use a fork to beat up your eggs, half-and-half, mustard, pepper, and salt in a cereal bowl.

Crumble two of the three slices of cooked bacon into the egg mixture. Now pour it over the scallions and scramble the whole thing up.

Put your eggs on a plate, crumble your last slice of bacon over it, and scatter the parsley over the whole thing. Then devour!

1 serving, with 414 calories, 32 g fat, 24 g protein, 6 g carbohydrate, 1 g fiber

Eggs Puttanesca

Puttanesca sauce is a wonderful pasta sauce loaded with olives, capers, and artichoke hearts. You can find it with the other pasta sauces in your grocery store. In this quick and easy but wonderful dish, you poach the eggs in this flavorful sauce.

>   1 cup puttanesca sauce
>   4 eggs
>   2 tablespoons grated fresh Parmesan cheese

In a medium skillet, heat your puttanesca sauce over medium-low heat. When it's simmering, break the eggs into the skillet and cover. Poach for 5–7 minutes or until the whites are set. Transfer the eggs to two plates with a slotted spoon, then spoon the sauce remaining in the skillet over them. Top with Parmesan and serve immediately.

2 servings, each with 221 calories, 14 g fat, 15 g protein, 9 g carbohydrate, 1 g fiber

Note: *Try poaching eggs in other sauces as well, such as Creole sauce or salsa topped with Monterey Jack.*

Eggs on a Bed of Mushrooms, Onions, and Chicken Livers

Either you like chicken livers or you don't. I adore them, and liver is the most nutritious food I know. So I came up with this recipe to give me yet another way to eat chicken livers and eggs. I liked it so much that I made it again the next day.

> 1 tablespoon butter
> 3 mushrooms, sliced
> ½ medium onion, sliced
> 1 clove garlic
> 2 chicken livers
> Salt and pepper to taste
> 3 eggs

Coat your medium skillet with nonstick cooking spray and put it over medium heat. Melt a third of the butter (a teaspoon or so) and start sautéing the mushrooms and onion together.

While that's happening, peel and crush your garlic and cut your chicken livers into bite-sized pieces. Remember to stir the mushrooms and onions.

When the onion is translucent and the mushrooms have softened and changed color, add another teaspoon of butter. Now stir in the garlic and the chicken livers. Sauté, stirring often, until the red is gone from the chicken livers, but there's still a little pink—nothing is worse than overcooked liver. Salt and pepper quickly. Now transfer the whole mixture to a serving plate and put a pot lid over it to keep it warm.

Wipe your pan quickly with a paper towel. (Don't burn yourself!) Spray it again, put it back on the heat, and throw in the last teaspoon of butter. Crack in your eggs. Cover the pan, let 'em fry for a few minutes, then uncover. Chances are that the tops of the whites will still be gooey. Add a teaspoon or two of water to the pan and re-cover it. The steam will cook the tops without your having to flip the eggs. Cook to your preferred degree of doneness. Use a pancake turner to transfer the eggs to your plate, right on top of the mushroom mixture. Salt, pepper, devour—and prepare to not be hungry again for a good 5 hours.

1 serving, with 417 calories, 27 g fat, 30 g protein, 12 g carbohydrate, 2 g fiber

Spinach-Mushroom Frittata

A frittata is an Italian omelet that doesn't need to be folded. This is a wonderful quick supper and a good choice if you have vegetarians over for dinner.

>   2 tablespoons butter
>   2 tablespoons olive oil
>   1 large onion, chopped
>   8 ounces sliced mushrooms
>   1 clove garlic, peeled and crushed
>   1 10-ounce package frozen chopped spinach, thawed
>   6 large eggs
>   ½ teaspoon pepper
>   ½ teaspoon salt
>   2 teaspoons brown mustard
>   1 teaspoon dried oregano
>   ¾ cup grated fresh Parmesan cheese
>   ¾ cup grated fresh Romano cheese

You'll need a big, heavy skillet with an ovenproof handle; I use my cast-iron skillet. Give it a shot of nonstick cooking spray and put it over medium heat. Add the butter and olive oil and swirl them together as the butter melts. Now add the onion and mushrooms and start sautéing them.

When the mushrooms are soft and the onion is translucent, quite a lot of liquid will have cooked out of them. Stir in the garlic, turn the heat to low, and let the whole thing simmer for a couple more minutes while you drain the spinach. Do drain it well! Easiest is to dump it into a strainer and press it hard with the back of a spoon. Then add the drained spinach to the mushrooms and onion and stir the whole thing together till everything is distributed evenly.

Break your eggs into a big bowl, preferably one with a pouring lip (a big measuring cup works well too), and add the pepper, salt, mustard, oregano, and ½ cup each of the Parmesan and Romano. Whisk everything together.

Stir the egg and cheese mixture over the veggies in the skillet. Spread everything into an even layer. Cover the skillet and cook over low heat for 12–15 minutes or until all but the very top is set. Turn on your broiler.

Sprinkle the reserved cheeses over the top. Now run the whole skillet under the broiler for 3–5 minutes, until the top is golden. Cut into wedges to serve.

6 servings, each with 270 calories, 20 g fat, 17 g protein, 7 g carbohydrate, 2 g fiber

Zucchini-Pepper Frittata

My charming neighbors, Keith and Peter, grow more vegetables on their half-acre lot than you could possibly believe. All summer long they pop over with wonderful garden surplus. I came up with this when their zucchinis were threatening to take over the neighborhood.

>   2 tablespoons olive oil
>   2 tablespoons butter
>   8 ounces zucchini, halved lengthwise and sliced thin
>   1 medium yellow bell pepper, diced
>   1 large onion, diced
>   2 cloves garlic, peeled and crushed
>   1 cup diced cooked chicken or turkey
>   8 eggs
>   2 tablespoons spicy brown mustard
>   1½ teaspoons Italian seasoning
>   3 tablespoons dry white wine
>   1½ cups shredded Muenster cheese

Give your big, heavy skillet a shot of nonstick cooking spray and place over medium heat. Add the olive oil and butter. When the butter is melted, add the veggies and garlic and sauté, stirring frequently, till the onion is translucent and the zucchini and pepper have softened a bit. Stir in the diced chicken and turn the burner to its lowest setting.

Crack the eggs into a great big glass measuring cup or a mixing bowl. Add the mustard, Italian seasoning, wine, and 1 cup of the cheese. Whisk everything together. Now pour the egg-and-cheese mixture over the veggies. Stir the whole thing just enough to make sure the egg mixture gets all the way to the bottom. Now cover the skillet and let your frittata cook for 15 minutes. It should be set, all except the very top. Turn on your broiler.

Scatter the last ½ cup of cheese over the top. Now run the skillet under the broiler, about 8 inches away, for about 5 minutes—until the top is golden brown. Cut into wedges to serve.

6 servings, each with 335 calories, 2 g fat, 22 g protein, 6 g carbohydrate, 1 g fiber

Breakfast Custard

You could have this for dessert, of course, but it has enough protein to serve as breakfast. How lovely would chilled lemon-vanilla custard be on a sultry summer morning? By the way, evaporated milk comes in 12-ounce cans and 5-ounce cans. So you want one of each.

> **17 fluid ounces evaporated milk**
> **4 large eggs**
> **⅓ cup Splenda**
> **1 teaspoon lemon extract**
> **½ teaspoon vanilla extract**
> **2 tablespoons vanilla whey protein powder**
> **Pinch salt**
> **1 teaspoon grated lemon zest**

Preheat the oven to 325°F. Spray a 1-quart casserole with non-stick cooking spray.

Simply whisk everything together. Pour into the prepared casserole.

Place a baking pan larger than your casserole in the oven. Put the casserole in the center of it. Now pour water into the baking pan, as deeply as you can without getting water into the casserole.

Bake for 1½ hours, or until a knife inserted in the center comes out clean. Remove from oven (it's safer to lift the casserole out of the water bath and let the water cool before moving the baking pan) and let the custard cool. Then chill overnight before serving.

4 servings, each with 284 calories, 15 g fat, 20 g protein, 17 g carbohydrate, trace fiber

Ham, Cheese, and Broccoli Egg Puff

You'll thank me for this the next time you have leftover ham in the house. And it reheats beautifully. Just cut a square and nuke it for a couple of minutes at 6 or 7 power. Makes a great quick breakfast!

6 eggs
1 cup cottage cheese
2 teaspoons prepared horseradish
1½ teaspoons dry mustard
¼ teaspoon salt or Vege-Sal
¼ teaspoon pepper
1½ cups small ham cubes
1 10-ounce package frozen chopped broccoli, thawed and drained
2 cups shredded cheddar cheese, regular or low-fat

Preheat the oven to 325°F. Spray an 8-inch square baking dish with nonstick cooking spray.

In a mixing bowl, whisk together the eggs, cottage cheese, horseradish, dry mustard, salt, and pepper.

Pour half the egg mixture into the prepared baking dish. Sprinkle the ham cubes in an even layer over the egg, then the broccoli in an even layer over that. Sprinkle the shredded cheese evenly over that, then pour the remaining egg mixture over the whole thing.

Bake for 50–60 minutes, or until puffed and turning golden. Cut into squares to serve.

9 servings, each with 218 calories, 14 g fat, 18 g protein, 4 g carbohydrate, 1 g fiber

Salmon and Asparagus Casserole

What an elegant Sunday brunch! Just as good on Monday too if you have leftovers. Just cut a square and nuke it at 6 or 7 power for a couple minutes in your microwave.

8 ounces salmon fillet
1 pound thin asparagus spears
6 eggs
1 cup cottage cheese
1½ tablespoons lemon juice
½ teaspoon lemon pepper
½ teaspoon salt or Vege-Sal
½ teaspoon dried dill or 2 teaspoons snipped fresh
8 ounces Swiss cheese slices

Preheat the oven to 350°F. Spray an 8-inch square baking pan with nonstick cooking spray.

If your salmon has skin, remove it. Now flake or chop it up. Reserve.

Snap the ends off your asparagus where it wants to break naturally. Lay it on your cutting board and cut it into ½-inch lengths. Reserve.

In a mixing bowl, preferably one with a pouring lip, whisk together the eggs, cottage cheese, and seasonings. Pour half of this mixture into the prepared baking pan.

Sprinkle the flaked salmon evenly over the egg mixture. Layer the asparagus over that, then lay the cheese slices evenly over that. Pour the rest of the egg mixture over the whole thing.

Bake for 50–60 minutes, till puffed and golden. Cut into squares to serve.

9 servings, each with 197 calories, 11 g fat, 20 g protein, 4 g carbohydrate, 1 g fiber

Strawberry Smoothie

Frozen fruit gives this the great frosty texture of a milk shake. Feel free to use any fruit—blueberries, blackberries, raspberries, frozen berry blend, frozen peach slices. You can freeze precut melon or pineapple chunks from the produce department to throw into smoothies. If you freeze bananas to use in your smoothies, cut them into a few chunks first to make them easier to blend.

> 1 cup plain yogurt
> ½ cup milk
> ½ cup unsweetened frozen strawberries
> 2 tablespoons vanilla whey protein powder
> 1 teaspoon to 2 tablespoons Splenda, or to taste
>   (feel free to use stevia—it's a lot sweeter than
>   Splenda)
> Guar or xanthan (optional, but makes it thicker)

Just throw everything into your blender and run it till it's smooth.

1 to 2 servings; assuming 1, each will have 375 calories, 14 g fat, 34 g protein, 22 g carbohydrate, 2 g fiber

Yogurt Parfait

This makes a great breakfast, but I like it as a bedtime snack too.

> **1 teaspoon vanilla extract (or do what I do and use a couple of capfuls)**
> **1 tablespoon Splenda, or to taste**
> **1 cup plain yogurt**
> **½ cup fruit—berries are great, as are sliced peaches or nectarines (use thawed unsweetened frozen fruit in the winter)**
> **¼ cup All-Bran, All-Bran Extra Fiber, or Fiber One cereal**

Do you really need instructions? Stir the vanilla and Splenda into the yogurt and add the fruit. Sprinkle the All-Bran over the whole thing and eat. (Taking lunch to work? Stir up the vanilla yogurt in a snap-top container and throw in frozen fruit, unthawed. Carry the All-Bran in a baggie. The fruit will keep the yogurt cold for several hours. When lunch rolls around, just add the All-Bran to the yogurt and fruit and devour.)

Assuming strawberries and regular All-Bran, 231 calories, 9 g fat, 11 g protein, 23 g carbohydrates, 7 g fiber

4

Baked Goods and
Other Grainy Stuff

Perhaps the hardest part of getting used to the glycemic-load diet is learning to live without grains. We've been told so often, for so long, that grains are good for us, that bread is the staff of life. We can understand intellectually why it's not so, why grains are the worst thing for us. Yet somehow it still feels wrong to pass them up.

For so many of us, grains are comfort food. All our lives we've been eating cereal for breakfast, a sandwich for lunch, chicken noodle soup when we have a cold, Mom's homemade bread, hot out of the oven. It's disorienting to give these foods up.

You'll get over it; I promise. As your waistline shrinks, as you feel better and better, as your energy level skyrockets, as your health improves, you'll get over it.

And Remember . . .

These baked goods have a low-glycemic load only if you eat them in moderation—one serving a day, no more. (That's one serving a day of *one* of these, not one of each!) *Glycemic load equals glycemic index times total grams of carbohydrate.* Eat too many grams of carbohydrate, even from these recipes, and you'll wind up with a high glycemic load.

Don't I Need Whole Grains?

In recent years we've been told that whole grains are incredibly beneficial, that the more of them we eat the healthier we'll be. But here's the thing: those studies compare people who eat whole grains to people who eat *refined grains*—grains with the fiber, vitamins, and minerals removed. I have yet to see one study that shows that people who eat lots of whole grains are healthier than people who *don't eat grains at all*.

My personal experience tells me Dr. Rob is right. When I tell people how disastrous a low-fat, high-carbohydrate diet was for me, people often respond, "Oh, but you need to eat *whole* grains." I reply that by 1995, when I dropped the grains from my diet, I hadn't bought white bread or white rice in more than fifteen years. Whole grains and other "healthy" starches got me up to nearly 200 pounds at five-foot-two, with borderline high blood pressure to boot.

Grains have been part of the human diet only since the Agricultural Revolution, about 10,000 years ago—a tiny fraction of

Dr. Rob Says: Whole Grains = Sugar Rocks with a Few Vitamins

There's no doubt that whole-grain bread and brown rice have more vitamins and fiber than white bread and white rice, but when it comes to raising your blood sugar, they're just as bad, even worse. Whole grains are packed solid with starch crystals. These little rocks turn to sugar as soon as they hit your digestive tract. Unless you're malnourished, you don't need the vitamins. There isn't enough fiber in them to do you any good. You certainly don't need the sugar shock.

our history. We all have hunter-gatherer ancestors—and hunter-gatherers don't eat grains. If grains were an essential part of human nutrition, our ancestors wouldn't have survived long enough to figure out farming and start eating them.

A Few Store-Bought Items

There are a few commercially made baked goods that fit into a low-glycemic-load diet. They manage this by having some of the starch replaced by fiber. Fiber is a carbohydrate, but you can't digest it, so it doesn't push up your blood sugar or trigger an insulin release.

- **Low-carb tortillas.** I mentioned these in Chapter 2—they're a great thing to keep on hand.
- **Low-carb bread.** True low-carb bread is getting harder and harder to find, but there are still a few brands out there. Read labels. At this writing, Trader Joe's carries low-carb whole-grain bread, Arnold Bakery lists a "carb-counting" bread on its website, and Healthy Life bakery lists a few varieties that have six grams of nonfiber carbohydrate per slice. My favorite low-carb bread has long been the Carb Conscious bread from Natural Ovens of Manitowoc; I've been ordering it from the website, naturalovens.com. Sadly, at this writing the company is unsure whether it will continue making the Carb Conscious bread, but it's certainly worth visiting the website to find out.
- **Fiber crackers.** Most crackers have not only a high glycemic load but trans fats as well. Bad stuff. But there are two brands of crackers I know of that are mostly wheat bran, Bran-a-Crisp and Fiber Rich. I haven't noticed a difference between the two; buy whichever you can find or comes cheaper. Fiber crackers are pretty boring on their own, but they make an agreeably crunchy base for cheese, liverwurst, pâté, or tuna salad.
- **All-Bran, All-Bran Extra Fiber, and Fiber One.** As I said in Chapter 2, these are the only cereals I know of that have a low-glycemic load. If you choose one of these for

breakfast, eat a protein food with it. These cereals also are good for making crumb crusts (see Chapter 12) and in yogurt parfaits.

Diluting the Starch

The trick to creating baked goods and other grain products with a low-glycemic load is to dilute the starch with a combination of fiber, protein, and fat. My recipes use bran, ground seeds and nuts, and protein powders to replace much of the flour. I've left just enough grain to get the familiar flavor and texture.

This means that this chapter, more than any other chapter in the book, will require you to lay in a stash of specialty ingredients. Your best bet for finding them all will be a good health food store.

About Baking Your Own Low-Carb Bread

I was torn about bread recipes. On one hand, good low-carb bread is hard to find. On the other hand, I included several bread machine recipes in *500 Low-Carb Recipes*, only to discover that many readers had a hard time getting them to rise.

I believe I've figured out the solution—at least, I hope I have. Here it is: When you make these recipes in your bread machine, do not simply put the ingredients in your bread machine, turn it on, and walk away. Instead, turn on the machine and let it knead the dough for three or four minutes. Then open the lid and look at your dough ball.

How does it look? Is it sticking to the sides of the bread case and "puddling" at the bottom? It's too wet. Add more of the dry ingredients (vital wheat gluten, flour, bran, protein powder) *one tablespoon at a time*. Sprinkle a tablespoon of one of those dry ingredients over the dough ball and let the machine knead it in before you decide whether you need more. If you do, add a little of the next dry ingredient—you're keeping your proportions right. When the dough forms a cohesive ball, it's right, and you can close the machine and walk away.

If you look at your dough ball and it's breaking into a couple of lumps instead of forming one ball, or if it's leaving dry flour behind, your dough is too dry. Sprinkle *one tablespoon* of water over the dough ball and let the machine knead it in. Repeat until you have a single cohesive ball that picks up all the flour. Then you can close the machine and walk away.

It's also good to know that the online low-carb stores carry low-carb bread machine mixes. A quick Web search will turn them up.

"Whole Wheat" Bread

The bran and germ give this bread a good wheaty flavor.

> 1 cup plus 2 tablespoons warm water
> 1 teaspoon salt
> 1 cup vital wheat gluten
> ½ cup wheat germ
> ½ cup wheat bran
> ¾ cup vanilla whey protein powder
> ⅔ cup whole wheat flour
> 2 tablespoons Sucanat
> 1 envelope active dry yeast

Put the water and salt in your bread machine first, then add everything else, with the yeast on top. Set your machine for its whole wheat cycle and follow the directions for making sure the dough ball is the right texture, then let it bake. Remove right away!

I got 18 slices; assuming you do too, each will have 128 calories, 2 g fat, 19 g protein, 9 g carbohydrate, 2 g fiber

Oatmeal-Marmalade Bread

This is my adaptation of the fantastic bread my mother used to make for the holidays—and when I say "fantastic," I mean it took the blue ribbon at the county fair. It's ambrosia toasted for breakfast.

1 cup boiling water
½ cup rolled oats
1 teaspoon salt
1 cup vital wheat gluten
¾ cup vanilla whey protein powder
½ cup flaxseed meal
⅔ cup whole wheat flour
1 tablespoon Sucanat
3 tablespoons low-sugar orange marmalade
1 tablespoon butter, melted
1 envelope active dry yeast

Put the boiling water and rolled oats in your bread maker's bread case and let them sit for about 30 minutes for the oats to soften.

Add the rest of the ingredients. Put all the dry stuff in first, making sure it completely covers the wet oats. Spoon the preserves into the corners, pour the melted butter around the edges, and sprinkle the yeast right on top. Turn the machine on, setting it for the whole wheat cycle. Follow the instructions earlier in the chapter for making sure the dough ball has the right texture, then run your machine through its whole wheat bread cycle. Remove from the bread case as soon as it's done baking. Serve with plenty of butter or toasted with cream cheese.

I get 15 slices; assuming you do too, each will have 189 calories, 6 g fat, 24 g protein, 12 g carbohydrate, 4 g fiber

Nadine's Miracle Bran Muffins

The best source of insoluble fiber in the American diet is the husk of the wheat kernel, that is, the bran. Unfortunately, most bran muffins are just cake; they don't provide enough fiber to do you any good. They're also full of flour and sugar. Dr. Rob and his nurse, Nadine, worked for two years to perfect a bran muffin that does the job. One muffin delivers more than 10 grams of fiber, as much as a bowl of All-Bran cereal. We like them best made with dried cranberries, but you can use apple chunks or blueberries or spice them up with grated fresh ginger. You can reduce the glycemic load further by substituting almond meal for whole wheat flour. The mashed yams—or sweet potatoes—are the key to a texture that makes these muffins better than cake.

1½ cups All-Bran cereal
1 cup whole wheat flour or almond meal
3 cups wheat bran
2 tablespoons brown sugar
1 teaspoon baking powder
1 teaspoon baking soda
1 teaspoon cinnamon
2 teaspoons ground allspice
½ teaspoon ground nutmeg
½ teaspoon salt
¾ cup dried cranberries
1 cup mashed canned yams or sweet potatoes
¾ cup chopped walnuts or almonds
4 eggs
1¼ cups milk
1 cup unrefined safflower oil
1 teaspoon vanilla extract
Butter for greasing the muffin cups

Adjust the oven rack to the lower-middle position. Preheat the oven to 350°F.

In a food processor with the S-blade in place, process the All-Bran until it has the texture of bread crumbs. Transfer to a large bowl. If you are using almond meal instead of flour, process the almonds until they have the texture of cornmeal.

Add the whole wheat flour (or the almonds) to the bowl along with the wheat bran, sugar, baking powder, baking soda, cinnamon, allspice, nutmeg, and salt. Stir to combine. Add the dried cranberries, yams, and walnuts.

Break the eggs into another large bowl and beat lightly with a fork. Add the milk, oil, and vanilla. Whisk to combine thoroughly.

Add about a third of the dry mixture to the egg-milk mixture and mix thoroughly. Repeat until all the ingredients are used.

Coat the muffin cups generously with butter. Spoon the batter into the muffin cups, filling to the rim. Bake until a toothpick inserted into the center of one of the muffins comes out clean or with a few moist particles adhering to it, about 20 minutes. Be careful not to overcook. Bran hardens if cooked too long.

12 muffins, each with 360 calories, 26 g fat, 10 g protein, 31 g carbohydrate, 11 g fiber (Use almond meal, and each will have 373 calories, 28 g fat, 13 g protein, 27 g carbohydrate, 9 g fiber)

Cinnamon, Flax, and Bran Granola

Dr. Rob hears from many people who have a little problem with, er, regularity when they first drop the grains from their diets. He asked me to come up with recipes to help them get bran and other fiber. This granola will do just that. It'll also keep you full and happy all morning long!

½ cup rolled oats
1 cup wheat bran
2 cups flaxseed meal
¾ cup wheat germ
½ cup shredded coconut meat
¾ cup oat bran
¼ cup vanilla whey protein powder
1½ teaspoons ground cinnamon
⅓ cup Splenda
⅛ cup Sucanat
¾ teaspoon salt
½ cup coconut oil, melted
¼ cup sugar-free pancake syrup or real maple syrup
2 tablespoons water
1½ teaspoons vanilla extract
½ cup chopped almonds
½ cup chopped pecans
½ cup chopped walnuts
½ cup shelled pumpkin seeds
½ cup sunflower seeds

Preheat the oven to 300°F. Line a big roasting pan with foil.

The easiest way to do this first part is with an electric mixer. Put everything from the rolled oats through the salt in a big bowl, and use the mixer to blend them till they're all distributed evenly.

Mix the melted coconut oil with the sugar-free pancake syrup, water, and vanilla extract.

Turn on your mixer and use it to slowly blend the liquid stuff into the dry stuff. Make sure everything is moistened evenly. Dump this mixture into your foil-lined roaster and use clean hands to press it out into an even layer. You want to compact it pretty well.

Slide the pan into the oven and bake it for 30 minutes. Pull the pan out and set it on a heatproof surface (like the top of your stove). Use a pizza cutter or a knife to cut the baked stuff into squares about ½ inch across. Stir the whole mass around, then spread it into a layer again. (You're not packing it down this time.) Spread the nuts and seeds on top and slide the pan back into the oven.

Continue roasting the granola for at least another 45 minutes, stirring it every 15–20 minutes. You want to make sure the flax mixture is dried thoroughly. When it's done, pull it out, let it cool, and store it in an airtight container.

Eat like any granola—serve it with milk or cream, stir it into yogurt, however you like.

18 ⅓-cup servings, each with 350 calories, 26 g fat, 15 g protein, 23 g carbohydrate, 13 g fiber

Hot "Cereal"

On a chilly winter morning, you'll thank me for this recipe. Not only does this have a low-glycemic load, but it has more protein than three eggs. It'll keep you going for hours!

½ cup flaxseed meal
½ cup almond meal
½ cup vanilla whey protein powder
¼ cup wheat bran
¼ cup oat bran
¼ teaspoon salt

Simply mix everything together and store in a snap-top container in your fridge or freezer. To prepare cereal, place ⅓ cup of the mixture in a bowl and stir in ⅓ cup of hot water. Let the mixture stand for a minute or so to thicken, then add milk or cream and the sweetener of your choice to taste. A little cinnamon is good too.

6 servings, each with 227 calories, 11 g fat, 25 g protein, 15 g carbohydrate, 8 g fiber

Flax Pancakes

These pancakes passed the acid test: I fed them to my six-year-old niece Halliday and nine-year-old nephew Henry, and they yummed them right down. No "These taste funny!" or "They're not like Mommy makes!" And my husband rated them a solid 10. All this, and each pancake has more protein than three eggs and nearly twice the fiber of a bowl of oatmeal, with only 4 grams of nonfiber carbohydrate.

> 1 cup flaxseed meal
> 1 cup vanilla whey protein powder
> ¾ teaspoon baking soda
> 1 tablespoon Splenda or Sucanat
> ½ teaspoon salt
> ¼ cup oat flour (you can leave this out if you want a
>   truly grain-free pancake)
> 1 teaspoon ground cinnamon
> 1 cup plain yogurt
> 2 eggs

In a mixing bowl, combine all the dry ingredients—everything from the flaxseed meal through the cinnamon—and stir well to combine.

Spray your biggest skillet (or a griddle) with nonstick cooking spray and put it over medium-high heat. (If your skillet or griddle has a good nonstick surface—mine does—you can skip the cooking spray.)

While the pan is heating, whisk the yogurt and eggs into the dry ingredients, making sure there are no pockets of dry stuff left.

When your skillet is hot enough that a drop of water will skitter across the surface, it's time to cook. Scoop the batter with a ¼-cup measure. Fry the first side until the edges look dry, then flip and cook the other side.

Serve with the topping of your choice; I like low-sugar jelly.

12 pancakes, each with 208 calories, 10 g fat, 21 g protein, 11 g carbohydrate, 7 g fiber

Note: You can find whole-grain oat flour at your health food store, or possibly in the baking aisle of your grocery store. In a pinch, run rolled oats through your food processor till they're finely ground.

Native American Flapjacks

Both corn and pumpkins are true American foods. Back when I was eating low fat, with lots of whole grains, I loved cornmeal pancakes—so I came up with these. They have enough cornmeal to give that great corn bread taste, with the protein and mineral kick from the pumpkin seeds.

⅔ cup whole-grain cornmeal
⅔ cup hulled pumpkin seeds (pepitas), ground
1 teaspoon salt
½ teaspoon baking soda
¼ cup vanilla whey protein powder
3 tablespoons butter, melted
2 cups plain yogurt
2 eggs

Combine all the dry ingredients in a mixing bowl. Stir them together till everything is distributed evenly.

In another bowl, whisk together the melted butter, yogurt, and eggs.

Put a big skillet or griddle, preferably with a nonstick coating, over medium-high heat. (If it doesn't have a nonstick coating, spray it well with nonstick cooking spray and add a little butter or oil between batches of cakes.) Let it get good and hot before you continue. Before you start cooking, your pan or griddle needs to be hot enough that a drop of water sprinkled on it skitters around the surface.

Skillet hot? Okay, let's cook. Dump the yogurt/egg mixture into the dry ingredients and stir the two together with a few swift strokes of your whisk—you want to stir just enough to make sure there are no pockets of dry stuff left.

Scoop the batter into the skillet with a ⅛-cup measure. Let each flapjack cook till the top surface looks dry before you flip 'em carefully. Let the other side brown, then serve with low-sugar jelly or sugar-free pancake syrup.

Makes 24, each with 60 calories, 3 g fat, 4 g protein, 4 g carbohydrate, 1 g fiber

Apple-Walnut Pancakes

These make a terrific weekend breakfast, and each pancake has as much protein as three eggs! Refrigerate the leftovers and warm them up for breakfast the rest of the week.

½ cup flaxseed meal
¾ cup vanilla whey protein powder
¼ cup Splenda
1¼ teaspoons baking powder
¼ teaspoon baking soda
1 teaspoon ground cinnamon
⅛ teaspoon ground allspice
¼ teaspoon ground nutmeg
⅛ teaspoon salt
2 small Granny Smith apples
1½ cups milk
2 eggs
3 tablespoons butter, melted
½ teaspoon blackstrap molasses
½ cup chopped walnuts

In a mixing bowl, stir all your dry ingredients together.

Quarter your apples, cut the cores out, and whack each quarter in two. Using your food processor with the S-blade in place, chop one of the apples pretty fine. Now add the second apple and continue chopping till *that* one is chopped fairly fine and the first one is even finer. (If you don't have a food processor, you could dice one apple quite small and grate the other. But that's a lot of work before breakfast.)

Pour your milk into another bowl. Stir the eggs, melted butter, and molasses into it.

At this juncture, put your biggest skillet or griddle over medium-high heat. I use my humongo-sized nonstick skillet. If you don't have a nonstick surface, give the sucker a coating of nonstick cooking spray.

Now dump the wet stuff into the dry stuff and whisk just until you're sure there are no pockets of dry stuff left.

Whisk in the chopped apples and walnuts.

When your skillet or griddle is hot, scoop the batter with a ⅓-cup measure. Cook until the edges are dry and the surface is losing its shiny look. Serve with butter. If you like, you can sprinkle a little cinnamon and Splenda on top, but it's really not essential.

10 pancakes, each with 242 calories, 14 g fat, 20 g protein, 12 g carbohydrate, 5 g fiber

Nutty Bran Crackers

Miss crackers? These are *so* worth your time.

> 2 cups hulled sunflower seeds
> ½ cup wheat bran
> ¼ cup walnuts
> ¼ teaspoon salt, plus extra for sprinkling
> 1½ teaspoons Sucanat
> ¼ teaspoon baking powder
> ¼ cup water

Preheat the oven to 350°F.

Dump the sunflower seeds into your food processor and use the S-blade to grind them to as fine a meal as you can get. Add the bran and walnuts and pulse till the walnuts are chopped too. Now add the salt, Sucanat, and baking powder and pulse to mix.

Turn on the processor and dribble the water in through the feed tube. Then turn off the processor.

Line a baking sheet with baking parchment. *(Do not skip the parchment! You will not be happy!)* Turn out the dough, form it into a cohesive ball, and put it in the middle of the parchment.

Tear off another sheet of parchment and put it over the dough ball. Flatten with your hand, then use your rolling pin to roll the dough out as thin as you possibly can—so long as there are no holes, the thinner, the better. I can make mine fill the whole big cookie sheet. (If your cookie sheets are kind of small, consider dividing the dough ball in two.)

Sprinkle lightly with salt and use a knife with a thin, straight blade to score it into squares the size of Wheat Thins.

Bake for 20 minutes or until golden brown. If they're underdone, they won't be crunchy. Feel free to transfer the ones that are brown to a cooling rack and return the underdone ones to the oven for another 5 minutes.

Cool on a wire rack and store in a container with a tight lid.

Makes 50 crackers, each with 38 calories, 3 g fat, 2 g protein, 2 g carbohydrate, 1 g fiber

Too-Good Cheese Crackers

Do you like cheese crackers? Why am I even asking? Everyone likes cheese crackers. These are the ultra-super-cheesy version. They're unbelievably flavorful.

> 8 ounces sharp cheddar cheese
> 1½ cups hulled sunflower seeds
> ½ teaspoon salt
> 2 teaspoons dry mustard
> ½ teaspoon paprika
> ½ teaspoon baking powder
> Pinch cayenne
> 2 tablespoons water

Preheat the oven to 350°F.

Using the shredding disk, grate the cheese in your food processor. Transfer the cheese to a bowl and swap out the shredding disk for the S-blade.

Put the sunflower seeds in the food processor and run until the sunflower seeds are ground to flour. Add the salt, mustard, paprika, baking powder, and cayenne and pulse to mix them into the sunflower flour.

Turn the food processor to "on" and add the shredded cheese through the feed tube a little at a time. By the time you've worked in all the cheese, the seed flour mixture will start forming a dough ball.

When all the cheese is worked in, add the water and run until it's worked in. Turn off the processor. Turn the dough out (scraping out any that adheres to the walls or blade of the processor) and divide into two equal balls.

Line a cookie sheet with baking parchment. *(Do not skip the parchment. You will be sorry. You have been warned.)* Put a dough ball in the center and cover it with another sheet of parchment. Using your hands, a rolling pin, or both (I use both), roll and press the dough out as thin as you can without holes. I can make half the dough cover a whole baking sheet. Keep it as even in thickness as you can.

Remove the top layer of parchment. Now use a knife with a thin, sharp blade to score the dough into crackers. Sprinkle lightly with a little extra salt if you want, but the cheese makes these plenty flavorful without.

Bake until the crackers are turning golden brown, about 15 minutes. If they're underdone, they won't turn crispy. When they're golden, transfer the whole parchment to a wire rack to cool. You may need to rescore the crackers to cut them apart (and, I warn you, some may break. They'll still taste amazing.)

If you have a second cookie sheet, start rolling and patting out the second dough ball while the first one bakes. (I can't find my second cookie sheet, darn it, so I have to wait till the first batch is done.) Either way, repeat the process with the second dough ball.

Store in a container with a tight lid for as long as they last, which won't be long.

I got about 80 crackers, each with 27 calories, 2 g fat, 1 g protein, 1 g carbohydrate, trace fiber

Sunflower-Cornmeal Cheese Crackers

These make a great snack, and they'd be killer with a bowl of chili or the Seriously Simply Southwestern Sausage Soup (see Chapter 7).

1 cup hulled sunflower seeds
⅓ cup whole-grain cornmeal
½ teaspoon ground cumin
¼ teaspoon cayenne
¼ teaspoon salt
2 cups shredded cheddar cheese
2 tablespoons water

Preheat your oven to 350°F.

In your food processor, using the S-blade, grind the sunflower seeds to a fine meal. Add the cornmeal, cumin, cayenne, and salt. Pulse to mix.

Turn the processor on and feed the cheese in, bit by bit. When it's all in, dribble in the water. Then stop the processor.

Line a cookie sheet with baking parchment. *(Do not skip the parchment. You have been warned—more than once.)* Turn the dough out onto the parchment—it will be crumbly but will stick together when you press it. Put another sheet of parchment over the dough. Using your hands and a rolling pin, coax the dough out to a thin, even, unbroken sheet—it should cover most of the cookie sheet. Peel off the top sheet of parchment.

Now use a knife with a sharp, thin blade to score the dough into squares the size of Wheat Thins.

Bake for 18 minutes and check. They should be browning a bit. If not, give 'em a few more minutes.

When your crackers come out of the oven, rescore them right away—they'll have melted together a bit. If the ones in the middle are still underdone, you can always transfer the ones that are done to a snap-top container and give the ones that are still soft another run into the oven. If they're underdone, they won't be crisp.

Keep in an airtight container. Way, way too tasty.

4 dozen crackers, each with 39 calories, 3 g fat, 2 g protein, 1 g carbohydrate, trace fiber

5

Snacks and Other Pickup Food

"What can I have for a snack?" The question is a sign of our processed-food-eating times. To our great-grandparents, a snack was an apple, a half a sandwich, the leftover drumstick from last night's chicken. But 21st-century Americans have been taught that a "snack" is something crunchy, salty, usually starchy, and comes out of a cellophane bag. (Starchy snacks are always salty. Why? Because without salt, starch is flavorless, of course.)

We've developed the habit of eating mindlessly for entertainment. How many times have you gone through a big bag of chips without thinking about it? I call it "the hand-to-mouth routine." There's a very simple reason we can do this: starchy stuff doesn't fill you up. You can eat it nearly forever without feeling nauseated.

Low-glycemic-load snacks are different: they're satisfying. This can require some retraining. Pay attention to your hunger. When you're actually hungry, eat. When you're full, *stop*. And don't eat again till you're hungry again. If you're bored, *do something*!

Here are some quick and easy snack ideas.

- **Fresh fruit of any kind.** Grab an apple, an orange, a plum, a peach—whatever's at hand. Most convenience stores have an apple or a banana somewhere.
- **Nuts.** Peanuts, mixed nuts, cashews, smoky-flavored almonds, all nuts are nutritious, healthful—and filling! They are also available at convenience stores and mini-marts.
- **Pumpkin seeds.** My favorite crunchy, salty snack! Most mini-marts have pumpkin seeds, salted in the shell. They're full of minerals, especially zinc. And the shells mean you have to eat them one by one, so one little bag lasts a long time.
- **Sunflower seeds.** A real nutritional powerhouse, sunflower seeds are available everywhere. If you crave variety, they come in interesting flavors like nacho cheese, ranch, and barbecue. Like pumpkin seeds, if you buy sunflower seeds in the shell you can snack on them for a long time, because you'll have to crack and eat them one by one.
- **Pork rinds.** Despite their reputation as the nadir of junk food, pork rinds have twice as much protein as fat. Very filling!
- **Yogurt.** I'm wary of the multicolored, heavily sugared varieties, some of which are nearly devoid of protein. But there's a wide variety of flavored yogurts in your grocer's dairy case, many sweetened with Splenda. Or do what Dr. Rob does: spoon plain yogurt into a dish with cut-up fruit. He says that often the fruit adds all the sweetness he needs, but that when he does want a touch more sweetness, ½ to 1 teaspoon is all the sugar he needs.
- **String cheese or other individually wrapped cheese bites.** An ounce or two of cheese will fill you up for hours.
- **Hard-boiled eggs.** Like cheese, hard-boiled eggs will keep you satisfied for a long time.
- **Beef jerky.** Available at truck stops and convenience stores everywhere.
- **Fiber crackers.** I said in Chapter 4 that most crackers have a high-glycemic load and are full of trans fats to boot. But if you look around, you can find fiber crackers, the only

crackers I know of with a really low-glycemic load. The two brands I see most often are Fiber Rich and Bran-a-Crisp, which I find at health food stores. These crackers consist largely of bran, glued together with a modest quantity of rye flour. Fiber crackers are pretty boring on their own, but with a little butter, peanut butter, or, my favorite, liverwurst, they're pretty good! Good with dips too.

- **Finn Crisp or Wasa Fiber Rye.** If you can't find fiber crackers, look for Finn Crisp or Wasa Fiber Rye. These flatbreads are crunchy and tasty and high in fiber. If you can limit yourself to just one or two, they shouldn't mess up your blood sugar.

The following recipes are great party foods, but you owe it to yourself to make them just for you and your family, should you have one. Turn to them anytime you want something delicious you can simply pick up and shove in your face.

Sweet and Spicy Punks

These are addictive! Luckily, they're also good for you.

> 1 egg white
> ⅓ cup Splenda or sugar
> 1 tablespoon chili powder
> 1 teaspoon ground cinnamon
> ½ teaspoon salt
> ¼ teaspoon ground cumin
> ¼ teaspoon cayenne, or more to taste
> 2 cups hulled pumpkin seeds (pepitas)

Preheat the oven to 350°F. Line a jelly roll pan or roasting pan with baking parchment.

Liberate your egg white from the yolk. (Feed the yolk to the dog; who needs to store an extra egg yolk in hopes that it'll be needed before it goes bad?) In a medium, fairly deep mixing bowl, whisk the white till it's frothy, but not whipped stiff.

Now whisk in the Splenda or sugar and all the seasonings.

Add half your pumpkin seeds and stir till they're coated. Add the second cup and stir again, till they're all evenly coated.

Spread your pumpkin seeds evenly on the parchment-lined pan. Stick 'em in the oven and set your timer for 5 minutes. When it goes off, stir your seeds, breaking them apart a bit as you do so. Put 'em back in and set the timer for another 5 minutes. Stir and separate again. Roast for a final 5 minutes or until the seeds are dry and browning a bit.

Pull 'em out of the oven, break up any clumps that are left, and let cool. Store in a snap-top container if you don't devour them all that day.

8 servings, each with 197 calories, 16 g fat, 9 g protein, 8 g carbohydrate, 2 g fiber

Curried Buttery Cashews

Oh. My. God. These are so good I made them in big batches and sent them to family for Christmas.

> 3 tablespoons butter
> 4 cups raw cashew pieces
> 2 teaspoons salt or 1 tablespoon Vege-Sal
> ½ teaspoon garlic powder
> ½ teaspoon onion powder
> ½ teaspoon paprika
> 1 teaspoon curry powder
> Pinch cayenne

Preheat the oven to 350°F. Put your butter in a big roasting pan and put it in the oven while it heats.

In a few minutes your butter should be melted. Pull the pan out of the oven, add the cashews, and stir until they're coated evenly with the butter. Return to the oven and roast for 10–12 minutes, stirring two or three times during the cooking.

While the cashews are roasting, stir together all the seasonings in a little dish.

When your cashews are a pretty gold color, pull 'em out of the oven. Sprinkle the seasonings over them and stir till they're coated evenly. Store in a container with a tight lid. Oh, who am I kidding? These will never stick around long enough to get stale!

20 servings, each with 166 calories, 14 g fat, 4 g protein, 8 g carbohydrate, 2 g fiber

Note: See those cashew pieces? You can use whole raw cashews if you like, and they'll look more impressive. But at my local health food store raw cashew pieces cost less than half of the whole ones, and they taste just as good as the whole ones.

Spiced Peanuts

These subtly spicy-sweet, Indian-inspired peanuts are very, very special.

> 2 tablespoons coconut oil
> 2 tablespoons ground coriander
> 1 tablespoon ground cumin
> 2 tablespoons Sucanat
> 2 teaspoons salt
> 6 cups unsalted dry-roasted peanuts
> 1 tablespoon dark sesame oil

Preheat the oven to 350°F. Put your coconut oil in a big roasting pan and put it in the oven while it heats.

Meanwhile, stir together your coriander, cumin, Sucanat, and salt.

Now pull out your roasting pan; your coconut oil will have melted. Dump your peanuts into the pan, add the sesame oil, and stir till the peanuts are coated evenly with the oils.

Sprinkle the seasoning mixture over the peanuts and stir till the peanuts are coated evenly.

Put the pan back in the oven and roast for 10 minutes, stir again, and roast for another 5–10 minutes. That's it!

24 servings, each with 235 calories, 20 g fat, 9 g protein, 9 g carbohydrate, 3 g fiber

Note: Most grocery stores carry jars of unsalted dry-roasted peanuts, but I get mine far cheaper in bulk at my health food store.

Tortilla Pizza

This is so easy you'd have thought of it yourself, but now you don't have to. I use Ragú's jarred pizza sauce. Feel free to add pepperoni, browned Italian sausage, sautéed bell pepper and onion, mushrooms, anchovies—whatever you like on your pizza. But this version is the quickest and easiest!

> 1 low-carb tortilla
> ½ teaspoon olive oil
> 1 tablespoon pizza sauce
> 1½ ounces shredded mozzarella cheese

Preheat your oven to 400°F.

Lay your tortilla on a cookie sheet. Brush it with a little olive oil. Spread the pizza sauce over that, then sprinkle the cheese over that. Bake for 10–12 minutes, till the cheese is melted and flecked with gold. Wait 5 minutes (if you can!) to let it cool a tad, then cut into quarters. Sprinkle with oregano, hot red pepper flakes, and/or grated Parmesan, as you like, and devour.

1–2 servings; assuming 1, each will have 216 calories, 15 g fat, 14 g protein, 14 g carbohydrate, 8 g fiber

Lemon-Mustard Wings

Tangy and garlicky.

> ¼ cup olive oil
> 2 tablespoons lemon juice
> 2 tablespoons brown mustard
> 2 teaspoons salt or Vege-Sal
> 1 teaspoon pepper
> 5 cloves garlic, peeled and crushed
> 2 pounds chicken wings

Whisk together everything but the wings.

Put your wings in a big resealable plastic bag and pour the marinade over them. Seal the bag, pressing out the air as you go. Turn the bag several times to make sure all the wings are coated evenly, then throw the bag in the fridge. Let 'em sit for at least an hour or two, turning the bag over if you should happen to open the fridge in the meantime.

When cooking time comes, arrange the wings on your broiler rack. Broil a good 6–8 inches from the heat, turning every 10–12 minutes, till golden crisp and cooked through. If you want, you can drain the marinade from the bag and use it to baste once or twice during the cooking period, but be sure to quit basting a good 5 minutes before they're done to give the heat time to kill the raw chicken germs!

Serve hot, with plenty of napkins.

4 servings, each with 270 calories, 23 g fat, 13 g protein, 3 g carbohydrate, trace fiber

Five-Spice Wings

Five-spice powder is a traditional Chinese spice blend. Find it in the international aisle of your grocery store. These are sweet and spicy!

1 tablespoon five-spice powder
1 tablespoon Sucanat
½ teaspoon garlic powder
1½ teaspoons salt or Vege-Sal
4 pounds chicken wings
2 tablespoons tomato sauce
2 tablespoons low-sugar apricot preserves
¼ cup chicken broth
2 tablespoons Splenda
2 teaspoons soy sauce
2 tablespoons apple cider vinegar
1 teaspoon grated fresh ginger
2 tablespoons peanut oil or olive oil

Preheat the oven to 375°F.

Mix together the five-spice powder, Sucanat, garlic powder, and salt or Vege-Sal.

Set aside 1 tablespoon of this mixture in a medium bowl. Sprinkle the rest evenly all over your wings. Lay the wings in a big roasting pan, skin side up, and slide them into the oven.

OK, grab that bowl with the set-aside seasoning mixture. Measure all the remaining ingredients into it and stir 'em up.

When your wings have been roasting for 15–20 minutes, baste them with the sauce you've made. Repeat about 15 minutes later and 15 minutes after that. By then your wings should be looking pretty done!

Serve the wings with the rest of the sauce for dipping.

8 servings, each with 184 calories, 12 g fat, 13 g protein, 4 g carbohydrate, trace fiber

Huevos El Diablo

Or, if you prefer, Mexican Deviled Eggs, though I invented them my very own self, right here in Indiana.

> 6 hard-boiled eggs
> 2 tablespoons canned diced green chilies
> 2 tablespoons mayonnaise
> 1 tablespoon sour cream
> ¼ teaspoon ground cumin
> ½ teaspoon chili powder
> Pinch cayenne, plus extra for garnish
> 2 tablespoons minced red onion
> 2 tablespoons minced fresh cilantro

Peel your eggs and then split each one lengthwise. Turn the yolks out into a mixing bowl and put the whites on a plate.

Using a fork, mash the yolks up as finely as you can. Then add the chilies, mayonnaise, and sour cream and mash again; you're trying to get the yolk mixture as creamy as you can.

Stir in the cumin, chili powder, and cayenne, mixing well to get the seasonings well distributed. Now add the minced onion and cilantro and stir again.

Stuff the yolk mixture back into the hollows of the whites. (If you really want to get fancy, you can use a pastry bag to pipe the yolk mixture in pretty rosettes, but I sure wouldn't bother.) Sprinkle a teeny bit of cayenne over the stuffed eggs for garnish and serve.

12 servings, each with 60 calories, 5 g fat, 3 g protein, 1 g carbohydrate, trace fiber

Christmas Party Stuffed Eggs

What with the red peppers and the green parsley, these look as festive as they taste. But don't take the name too literally; they'll be welcome any time of year.

6 hard-boiled eggs
¼ cup light mayonnaise
1½ teaspoons lemon juice
½ teaspoon chicken bouillon concentrate
3 slices cooked bacon, crumbled fine
⅛ teaspoon pepper
2 dashes Tabasco sauce
⅛ teaspoon soy sauce
1½ teaspoons minced scallion
1½ teaspoons minced drained roasted red pepper
    jarred in water
1½ teaspoons minced fresh parsley
Paprika (optional)

Peel your eggs, slice 'em in half lengthwise, and turn the yolks into a mixing bowl. Put the whites on a plate and set aside.

Mash the yolks thoroughly with a fork. Add the mayonnaise, lemon juice, and chicken bouillon concentrate and mash again, stirring well until the yolks are creamy and the bouillon concentrate is completely dissolved.

Now stir in everything else except the paprika. Stuff the yolk mixture back into the whites. Garnish with a sprinkle of paprika if you really want to, but they're pretty and very flavorful without it.

12 servings, each with 60 calories, 4 g fat, 4 g protein, 1 g carbohydrate, trace fiber

Mustard-Horseradish Beef Roll-Ups

Easy and pretty.

    3 tablespoons mayonnaise
    3 tablespoons brown mustard
    1 tablespoon prepared horseradish
    1 scallion, minced
    1 roasted red pepper, jarred in water, drained
    8 ounces deli roast beef, sliced medium-thick
    6 ounces shredded Monterey Jack cheese
        (about 1½ cups)

Mix together the mayonnaise, mustard, horseradish, and minced scallion. Slice your roasted red pepper lengthwise into as many strips as you have slices of beef.

Lay a slice of roast beef on your cutting board. Spread it with the mustard/mayo mixture and sprinkle it all over with shredded cheese. Now lay a strip of roasted red pepper across one end of the whole thing, and roll up your slice of roast beef around it. Place on a plate, seam side down. Repeat until you're out of everything. (Unless you're better at this than I am, you may not come out exactly even. *C'est la guerre.*)

Chill your beef rolls for several hours. Right before serving, cut each one across into five or six rolls about 1 inch long. Pierce them with toothpicks, arrange them prettily on a lettuce-lined plate, and serve.

24 servings, each with 58 calories, 4 g fat, 5 g protein, 1 g carbohydrate, trace fiber

6

Side Dishes and Side-Dish Salads

Dropping potatoes, rice, and noodles from your diet can be disorienting. Sure, steak, chicken, chops, and the like are friendly and familiar. But what goes on that third of the plate where the starch used to be?

Vegetables! But not just plain buttered vegetables (although they're fine). Interesting vegetables. Heck, exciting vegetables, both hot and cold. It's time to broaden your repertoire of vegetable dishes and salads. Here are enough ideas for you to get a great start!

Side Dishes

There are a couple of foundation recipes you need first. Just as there are thousands of recipes for potatoes or rice, these basic recipes lend themselves to endless variations. And not only do they have a low-glycemic load and far more nutrients than your old starchy favorites, but they cook faster too. Both recipes are based on cauliflower. So instead of grabbing a sack of potatoes every time you go to the grocery store, grab a couple of heads of cauliflower!

This first foundation recipe is an old standard in the low-carb community. It's a stand-in for mashed potatoes. Even if you're sure you don't like cauliflower, try it. More than once, I've served a guest "fauxtatoes" topped with a flavorful gravy, only to have him or her yum down five or six mouthfuls before looking up, puzzled, to say, "Wait. Those aren't mashed potatoes . . . What *are* they?" They never guess it's cauliflower.

Fauxtatoes

These are remarkably good just as they are and fabulous with gravy. Try melting in a little cream cheese if you want a richer texture.

½ head cauliflower
2 tablespoons butter, or to taste
Salt and pepper to taste

Fast and easy! Trim the leaves and the very bottom of the stem off your cauliflower and whack the rest into chunks. Put 'em in a microwavable casserole with a lid, add a few tablespoons of water, and cover. Nuke for 10–12 minutes or until tender.

When your cauliflower is cooked, drain it well. Use your blender, food processor, or stick blender to puree the cauliflower. Melt in the butter, add salt and pepper to taste, and serve.

3–4 servings; assuming 3, each will have 92 calories, 8 g fat, 2 g protein, 5 g carbohydrate, 2 g fiber

Cauliflower-Potato Mash

Want something a little more potatoey? The addition of just a little potato makes your pureed cauliflower a truly convincing mashed potato clone—with a vastly lower glycemic load and fewer calories and more vitamins to boot!

> ½ head cauliflower
> 5 ounces potato
> 2 tablespoons butter
> Salt and pepper

Trim the leaves and the very bottom of the stem off your cauliflower and whack it into chunks. Scrub or peel your potato and whack it into chunks. Put both in a microwavable casserole with a lid. Add a tablespoon or two of water, cover, and nuke on high for 12–15 minutes, or until both are good and tender.

Drain the veggies. Now use your blender, stick blender, or food processor to puree the two together. (I use my stick blender and puree the whole thing in the bowl I plan to serve it in.)

Stir in the butter and salt and pepper to taste and serve.

4 servings, each with 97 calories, 6 g fat, 2 g protein, 10 g carbohydrate, 2 g fiber

Note: Whether you make Fauxtatoes or Cauliflower-Potato Mash, feel free to play with the recipe. Anything you'd put in mashed potatoes—garlic, cheese, horseradish, you name it—is good in these purees.

Cauliflower "Rice"

Here is the second foundation recipe. Credit where credit is due: I first found this idea in Fran McCullough's wonderful book *The Low-Carb Cookbook*. I've used it literally hundreds of ways since, in everything from fried "rice" to "rice" salads.

This is the basic version. Butter, salt, and pepper it, if you like, or use it as a bed for a stir-fry.

½ head cauliflower

Trim the leaves and the very bottom of the stem from your cauliflower. Whack the rest into pieces that'll fit into the feed tube of your food processor.

Fit your food processor with its shredding disk. Now run the cauliflower through the shredding blade. Put the resulting cauliflower "rice" in a microwavable casserole with a lid. Add a couple of tablespoons of water and nuke on high for just 6–7 minutes. Uncover as soon as the microwave beeps to avoid overcooking. It's all about the texture here!

3 servings, each with 24 calories, trace fat, 2 g protein, 5 g carbohydrate, 2 g fiber

Rice-a-Phony

Here's a simple example of how to use cauliflower "rice." There's a basic principle here that you should pay attention to: the use of bouillon concentrate to flavor the "rice." Real rice is often cooked in broth, but this won't do for cauliflower rice since it doesn't absorb liquid. Stirring in bouillon concentrate gives us the flavor of broth without the water.

My brother John is a longtime Rice-a-Roni fan, especially the chicken-almond variety, so he loved this; he's the one who gave it this name. He was very surprised to learn that it contained no grain at all!

> ½ head cauliflower
> 2 teaspoons butter
> ¼ cup slivered almonds
> 1 bunch scallions, including the crisp greens, sliced
> ¼ cup chopped fresh parsley
> 2 teaspoons chicken bouillon concentrate

Do the cauliflower "rice" thing—trim your cauliflower, chunk it, run it through the shredding disk of your food processor, and microwave-steam the resulting cauliflower "rice" for 6 minutes.

Meanwhile, put your big, heavy skillet over medium heat, add the butter, and start sautéing the almonds in it.

OK, the almonds are golden, and the microwave has beeped. Drain the cauliflower and dump it into the skillet with the almonds. Stir in everything else, mixing till the chicken bouillon concentrate is dissolved and everything is well distributed. You're done!

3–4 servings; assuming 3, each will have 124 calories, 9 g fat, 5 g protein, 8 g carbohydrate, 3 g fiber

Note: For a nice variation, try pine nuts in place of the almonds.

Lemon-Garlic "Rice"

Great with take-out Greek chicken!

½ head cauliflower
3 tablespoons butter
4 large garlic cloves, peeled and crushed
1 lemon
½ cup dry white wine
2 teaspoons chicken bouillon concentrate
½ cup chopped fresh parsley

Trim the leaves and the very bottom of the stem from your cauliflower. Whack it into chunks and run them through the shredding disk of your food processor. Dump the resulting " rice" into a microwavable casserole with a lid, add a couple of tablespoons of water, cover, and nuke on high for 6 minutes.

Put your big, heavy skillet over low heat and start melting the butter. Add the crushed garlic cloves and sauté them slowly, without browning, for 5 minutes or so.

Meanwhile, grate the zest from your lemon and squeeze the juice. After the 5 minutes of sautéing time, add both to the garlic, along with the wine. Turn the heat up to medium and let the mixture simmer.

Your microwave has beeped by now! Pull out your "rice" and uncover it to keep it from turning to mush. Drain it too.

When the garlic-lemon-wine mixture has cooked down to half its original volume, stir in the chicken bouillon concentrate. When it's dissolved, add the "rice" and mix everything together well.

Stir in the parsley and serve.

3 servings, each with 150 calories, 12 g fat, 1 g protein, 5 g carbohydrate, 1 g fiber

Pecan "Rice"

With a good broiled steak and a glass of red wine, this makes for a glorious dinner. For that matter, if you have leftover steak or roast beef in the house, you could dice it and stir it into this rice dish for a skillet supper.

½ head cauliflower
¼ cup chopped pecans
1 bunch scallions
1 tablespoon butter
1 tablespoon olive oil
½ cup frozen peas
⅓ cup cooked wild rice
2 teaspoons beef bouillon concentrate
¼ cup dry white wine
Tabasco sauce to taste (start with a few dashes)
Salt and pepper to taste
¼ cup chopped fresh parsley

Trim the leaves and the very bottom of the stem from your cauliflower. Whack your cauliflower into chunks and run it through the shredding disk of your food processor. Dump the resulting "rice" into a microwavable casserole with a lid, add a tablespoon or two of water, cover, and nuke on high for 6 minutes.

Meanwhile, chop your pecans, spread 'em on a shallow baking pan, and run 'em into a 350°F oven for 10 minutes to toast. Set the timer, or you'll forget them, sure as you're born. (If you like, buy toasted salted pecans and just chop 'em. I promise not to tell.)

Slice your scallions, including the crisp part of the green.

Give your biggest skillet a shot of nonstick cooking spray and put it over medium-low heat. Add the butter and olive oil.

When the microwave beeps, pull out your cauliflower and uncover it to stop the cooking. Put your peas in a small dish, add a tablespoon of water, cover, and give 'em just 90 seconds to 2 minutes on high in the microwave.

OK, time to start combining stuff. Drain your cauliflower and dump it into the skillet. Add the wild rice, beef bouillon concentrate, and wine and stir everything up really well. Now give it a shot of the Tabasco and taste. Add more if it needs it. Let the whole thing cook together for 5 minutes to let the wine cook down a bit.

Meanwhile, drain your peas and throw 'em in; then salt and pepper the whole thing.

Right before serving, stir in the parsley and those toasted pecans. Serve and listen to the raves.

5 servings, each with 131 calories, 9 g fat, 3 g protein, 9 g carbohydrate, 3 g fiber

Note: *Look for teeny boxes of wild rice with the other rice in your grocery store. Don't buy "wild and long-grain rice blend." All the grains should be dark brown. Cook according to package directions and stash it in a snap-top container in your freezer. Then you'll have wild rice on hand whenever you want it!*

Parmesan Broccoli

Wonderful. You could use fresh broccoli, but you'd have to cut it up and blanch it—cook it in boiling water for just a few minutes—then drain it, before you could stir-fry it. After blanching, it would be very much like thawed frozen broccoli. So why work that hard?

> 2 tablespoons olive oil
> 1 pound frozen broccoli "cuts," thawed
> 1 clove garlic, peeled and crushed
> 1 teaspoon hot red pepper flakes
> 3 tablespoons grated Parmesan cheese—the cheap kind in the green shaker is fine
> ¼ teaspoon salt

Put your big, heavy skillet over high heat and add the olive oil. When it's hot, add the broccoli. Stir-fry it till it's tender-crisp, with a few brown spots.

Stir in the garlic and red pepper flakes and stir-fry for another minute or two.

Stir in the Parmesan and salt and serve.

3 servings, each with 143 calories, 11 g fat, 6 g protein, 8 g carbohydrate, 5 g fiber

Broccoli with Cashews

This fast and delicious Asian-style broccoli is far easier than it tastes.

> **1 pound broccoli**
> **2 tablespoons butter**
> **1½ teaspoons Sucanat**
> **2 tablespoons soy sauce**
> **1½ teaspoons rice vinegar**
> **1 clove garlic, minced**
> **⅛ teaspoon chili garlic paste**
> **¼ cup roasted salted cashews**

Cook your broccoli tender-crisp—you've probably gathered by now that I'd use frozen broccoli and microwave-steam it.

While your broccoli is cooking, melt the butter in a small saucepan and whisk in everything else but the cashews. Chop the cashews.

When your broccoli is tender-crisp and brilliant green, drain it and toss with your sauce. Add the cashews and toss again, then serve.

3 servings, each with 174 calories, 13 g fat, 5 g protein, 12 g carbohydrate, 4 g fiber

Stir-Fried Snow Peas with Water Chestnuts and Cashews

If you like Chinese food, you'll love this.

  3 cups fresh snow pea pods
  2 tablespoons peanut oil
  2 cloves garlic, minced
  1 tablespoon grated fresh ginger
  1 8-ounce can sliced water chestnuts, drained
  ¼ teaspoon chili garlic paste
  1½ teaspoons soy sauce
  ¼ cup roasted cashews, chopped

Pinch the ends off the snow peas and pull the strings off the sides. Have everything else prepped and standing by before you start cooking.

Put a big skillet or wok over high heat. When it's hot, add the peanut oil, then the snow peas, garlic, and ginger. Stir-fry till the snow peas are just barely tender-crisp. Stir in the drained water chestnuts, chili paste, and soy sauce and continue stir-frying till the water chestnuts are heated through. Stir in the cashews and serve.

3 servings, each with 212 calories, 14 g fat, 4 g protein, 19 g carbohydrate, 4 g fiber

Chipotle Mushrooms

You think simple sautéed mushrooms are good on a steak or in an omelet? Try these: unreal.

> 2 tablespoons olive oil
> 8 ounces sliced mushrooms
> ½ medium onion, chopped
> 2 cloves garlic, minced
> 1 chipotle chili canned in adobo, minced
> 2 tablespoons minced fresh cilantro
> Salt and pepper to taste

Put your big, heavy skillet over medium heat and add the olive oil. When hot, throw in the mushrooms, onion, garlic, and chipotle. Sauté, stirring often, for 8 or 9 minutes, until the mushrooms and onion are soft.

Stir in the cilantro and salt and pepper to taste and serve.

3 servings, each with 109 calories, 9 g fat, 2 g protein, 6 g carbohydrate, 2 g fiber

Blue Cheese Mushrooms

I came up with this from what I had in the fridge and served it smothering a pan-broiled rib-eye. Fantastic—and fantastically easy! But it would be equally good over a chicken breast, in an omelet, or on the side with almost anything.

2 teaspoons olive oil
2 teaspoons butter
8 mushrooms (about 4 ounces), sliced
1 medium onion, sliced
2 cloves garlic, peeled and crushed
2 tablespoons crumbled blue cheese
Seasoned salt to taste
Pepper to taste
4 dashes Tabasco sauce
¼ cup chopped fresh parsley

In a big skillet over medium heat, combine the olive oil and butter, swirling them together as the butter melts. Throw in the mushrooms, onion, and garlic.

Sauté until the onion is starting to brown and the mushrooms have softened and changed color. Add the blue cheese and stir till it's mostly melted in. Stir in the seasonings and serve.

2–4 servings, depending on what you serve with it; assuming 2 servings, each will have 150 calories, 11 g fat, 4 g protein, 10 g carbohydrate, 2 g fiber

Glad Zukes!

These Greek-style zucchini-feta pancakes make a great light meal all on their own. But they're also a killer side dish with roast lamb.

> **1 pound zucchini**
> **1 teaspoon salt or Vege-Sal, plus ¼ teaspoon (optional)**
> **½ small onion, minced**
> **1 clove garlic, peeled and crushed**
> **2 teaspoons dried oregano**
> **3 eggs**
> **¼ teaspoon pepper**
> **1 cup crumbled feta cheese**
> **⅓ cup rice protein powder**
> **3 tablespoons oat bran**
> **About ½ cup olive oil**

Shred your zucchini, with either your food processor's shredding disk or your box grater. Put the shreds in a bowl and sprinkle with ½ teaspoon of the salt. Stir the salt in. Now repeat with another ½ teaspoon salt, also stirring that in well. Let your salted zucchini sit for at least an hour, and all day is fine. (Obviously, you'll want to refrigerate it if you're letting it sit all day.)

Whenever you want to make your Glad Zukes!, dump your zucchini into a strainer. Press it with the back of a spoon to get out as much water as you can.

Put the zucchini into a mixing bowl and add the onion, garlic, oregano, eggs, ¼ teaspoon salt if you're using it, and pepper. Stir everything together well. Stir in the feta.

Now stir in the rice protein and oat bran. (You can substitute ½ cup of whole wheat flour if you absolutely must.)

Spray your biggest heavy skillet with nonstick cooking spray (not necessary if the skillet's nonstick) and place over medium-high heat. Add enough olive oil to cover the bottom of the skillet to about the depth of a dime. Let the oil get hot before you start frying your Glad Zukes!

Scoop your batter using a ¼-cup measure—you'll have to fry in three or four batches. Let the pancakes get good and brown on the bottom before flipping, or they'll fall apart when you do. Brown well on both sides and serve. These don't need a darned thing!

8 servings, each with 249 calories, 20 g fat, 14 g protein, 6 g carbohydrate, 1 g fiber

Green Beans and Portobellos Vinaigrette

My husband, not a mushroom fan, still gave these beans an A+ score. Quick, easy, and elegant.

2 tablespoons olive oil
1¾ pounds frozen green beans, thawed
1 cup chopped portobello mushroom caps
1 clove garlic, peeled and crushed
3 tablespoons sherry vinegar
Salt and pepper to taste

Put your big, heavy skillet over medium-high heat and add the olive oil. Slosh it around to cover the bottom of the skillet. Now add the green beans and chopped portobellos. Sauté, stirring often, till the beans are crisp-tender—8–10 minutes.

Stir in the garlic and vinegar and let the whole thing cook for another 3–5 minutes. Salt and pepper and serve.

6 servings, each with 88 calories, 5 g fat, 3 g protein, 11 g carbohydrate, 4 g fiber

Green Beans with Pine Nuts

A great change from the traditional almonds.

> 2 pounds green beans, fresh or frozen
> 1 clove garlic, peeled and crushed
> 2 tablespoons olive oil
> ¼ cup pine nuts
> 1 tablespoon butter

If you're using fresh beans, trim the ends and cut them into 2-inch lengths. If using frozen, simply start cooking them. Either way, put your beans in a microwavable casserole with a lid. Add a couple of tablespoons of water, cover, and microwave until just done through but still slightly crisp—10–12 minutes. Stir halfway through that time.

While the beans are steaming, crush your garlic and put it in a small cup. Pour the olive oil over it and let it sit.

Put your pine nuts in a dry skillet and stir over medium-low heat until they're touched with gold.

When your beans are done, drain them well. Toss with the garlic and olive oil and butter until the butter is melted. Stir in the pine nuts and serve.

8 servings, each with 98 calories, 7 g fat, 3 g protein, 8 g carbohydrate, 4 g fiber

Orange-Hazelnut Green Beans

Perfect for a holiday—or a weeknight, for that matter.

> 4 cups frozen crosscut green beans
> 4 teaspoons butter
> ¼ cup chopped hazelnuts
> 1 teaspoon grated orange zest
> 6 tablespoons orange juice
> 1 teaspoon rice vinegar or white wine vinegar

Start steaming your beans—I do mine for 7–8 minutes in the microwave, but a stovetop steamer is fine too.

Meanwhile, melt your butter over medium heat in a small, heavy skillet. Add your hazelnuts and sauté until they're golden.

Stir in the orange zest, juice, and vinegar. Simmer for just a minute or two, to cook down the sauce and intensify the flavor.

When your beans are tender but still bright green, toss with the sauce and serve.

4 servings, each with 131 calories, 9 g fat, 3 g protein, 13 g carbohydrate, 4 g fiber

Grilled Asparagus

You'll be surprised at how good this is!

1 pound fresh asparagus
2 tablespoons olive oil
Salt and pepper to taste

Preheat your electric tabletop grill.

Snap the ends off of your asparagus where the spears break naturally. Put them in a flat pan and toss them with the olive oil till they're coated. Sprinkle with salt and pepper.

Lay your spears across your hot grill, close the lid, and let cook for 4–5 minutes—until there are brown grill marks on the asparagus—and serve. This doesn't need any embellishment!

3–4 servings; assuming 3, each will have 114 calories, 9 g fat, 3 g protein, 7 g carbohydrate, 3 g fiber

Italian Asparagus

Unusual and wonderful.

> 2 pounds asparagus
> 3 tablespoons olive oil
> 2 cloves garlic, peeled and crushed
> ¼ cup capers, chopped fine
> 2 hard-boiled eggs, peeled and grated on the large holes of your box grater
> ¼ cup grated Romano cheese

Snap the ends off your asparagus where they break naturally. Cut into 1-inch lengths—I like to cut on the diagonal.

Give your biggest skillet a squirt of nonstick cooking spray (unless it's nonstick; then skip it) and put over medium-high heat. Add the olive oil. When the oil is hot, add the asparagus and stir-fry until it's brilliant green and crisp-tender.

Add the garlic and stir-fry for another minute or so; then stir in the chopped capers.

Pile the asparagus into bowls or onto plates. Top each serving with grated egg and Romano and serve.

4 servings, each with 186 calories, 15 g fat, 8 g protein, 6 g carbohydrate, 3 g fiber

Orange-Glazed Carrots

Good ol' carrots. They're cheap year-round and always available. They're usually part of the steamed vegetables that come on the side at restaurants. We love them, but they can get a little . . . boring. Well, forget that! These carrots are outstanding. So sweet and tasty they're almost a dessert.

> 1 pound carrots
> ¼ cup chopped pecans
> 1 orange
> 1 tablespoon butter
> 1 tablespoon dark rum
> 4 teaspoons Splenda and ½ teaspoon
>   blackstrap molasses *or* 4 teaspoons Sucanat

Preheat the oven to 350°F.

Peel your carrots and cut them into strips or slices, whatever you prefer—we like thin strips. Put them in a microwavable casserole with a lid, add a couple of tablespoons of water, cover, and nuke on high for 10 minutes.

OK, your oven is hot. Spread your pecans in a roasting pan and slide them in. Set the timer for 10 minutes.

Grate the orange's zest and squeeze the juice into a saucepan big enough to hold your carrots. Put on the stove over medium-low heat and add everything else. Stir together till this sauce is cooked down a little and getting syrupy.

By now your carrots should be done. Pull them out of the microwave, drain them, and dump them into the saucepan. Stir till the carrots are coated with the sauce.

Your pecans are toasted! Remove them from the oven, stir them into the carrots, and serve.

4 servings, each with 146 calories, 8 g fat, 2 g protein, 16 g carbohydrate, 4 g fiber

Parmesan Brussels Sprouts

I used to think I didn't like brussels sprouts, but that was because I'd had them only boiled and buttered. I've discovered I like them almost any way *other* than that. Slicing them, as in this recipe, turns them into a different vegetable.

> 1 pound brussels sprouts
> 1 tablespoon butter
> 1 tablespoon olive oil
> 1 clove garlic
> 1 tablespoon lemon juice
> 2 tablespoons grated fresh Parmesan cheese

Trim the bottoms of your brussels sprouts and remove any bruised or browned leaves. Now run 'em through your food processor using the slicing disk.

Put your big skillet over medium heat and throw in the butter and olive oil. Swirl them together as the butter melts. Now throw in the sliced brussels sprouts and start sautéing them.

While that's happening, peel and crush the garlic. Throw it in with the brussels sprouts. Keep sautéing, stirring often, until the sprouts are getting tender. You want them to brown some—the flavor this adds is really wonderful.

Stir in the lemon juice and Parmesan and serve.

4 servings, each with 113 calories, 7 g fat, 5g protein, 10 g carbohydrate, 4 g fiber

Side Salads

You're clear that salad is good for you? Good. Few things can do more for your health than serving a big salad at every dinner.

I'm going to assume you know how to make a basic tossed salad, though I will make a few points:

- Salad dressing is astonishingly easy to make and—like everything else—tastes better when you make it yourself.

The basic proportions for a vinaigrette dressing are two to three parts olive oil to one part vinegar, lemon juice, or a combination of the two. You can add a clove of garlic to this, or a squirt of mustard, a dash of oregano or Italian seasoning, a pinch of sugar or Splenda, a few drops of hot sauce. Of course a little salt and pepper is good. If you want a creamy dressing, add a dollop of mayonnaise. The variations are infinite, but the basics are unchanging.

- Be wary of fat-free bottled dressings. Many of them replace oil with corn syrup, which makes them sugary liquids! Furthermore, studies show that if you eat salad without fat, you don't absorb the antioxidants. Stick with oil-based dressings.
- Unless your family has violently differing opinions on salad dressings, do toss your salad with the dressing instead of simply pouring it on top of individual servings. It really improves the final product. Toss the salad with the dressing right before serving, or it will become soggy.
- If you want something crunchy in your salad, go for sunflower seeds or slivered almonds instead of croutons. Or try this: spray a microwavable plate with nonstick cooking spray. Now spread a handful of shredded Parmesan or Romano on it—this must have no additives or the trick won't work, so read the label. Microwave your plate of cheese for a minute to a minute and a half. When it cools, it'll be crisp. Crumble into your salad for a great cheesy crunch!

So go ahead, make a salad! Whether you cut up a dozen different ingredients or simply toss some bagged salad with bottled dressing, it's the best way to start a meal.

When you tire of simple green salad, try these.

Strawberry Salad

This salad looks as good as it tastes. And between the berries, the greens, and the almonds, it's ridiculously good for you. Make the dressing right before making the salad since its flavors are most vibrant when fresh.

> 6 tablespoons slivered almonds
> 4½ quarts mixed greens
> Strawberry Vinaigrette (recipe follows)
> 30 strawberries, sliced
> 1½ cups sliced celery from the pale inner heart
> 6 scallions, including the crisp greens, sliced

Toast your slivered almonds: just stir 'em in a dry skillet over medium heat till they're touched with gold.

Dump your mixed greens into a huge bowl—I use bagged mixed baby greens or Italian blend. Pour on the dressing and toss. Pile the salad on six plates or into six bowls.

Top with the strawberries, celery, scallions, and almonds. Serve immediately.

6 servings, each with 307 calories, 24 g fat, 8 g protein, 22 g carbohydrate, 10 g fiber

Strawberry Vinaigrette

20 strawberries
½ cup olive oil
½ cup balsamic vinegar
4 teaspoons Dijon or spicy brown mustard
1 teaspoon pepper
¼ cup Splenda (or sugar, if you must!)

Just assemble everything in your food processor (with the S-blade in place) or blender and run it till the strawberries are pureed. Best used fresh.

6 servings, each with 182 calories, 18 g fat, 1 g protein, 6 g carbohydrate, 1 g fiber

Coleslaw

Feel free to use bagged coleslaw mix if you don't feel like shredding your own cabbage.

> ½ head cabbage, shredded
> ¼ medium red onion, minced
> ⅓ cup light mayonnaise
> ⅓ cup plain yogurt
> 1 teaspoon brown mustard
> 1 tablespoon apple cider vinegar
> 1 teaspoon Splenda or sugar
> ⅛ teaspoon salt or Vege-Sal, or to taste

Pretty darned simple: Throw the cabbage and onion into a big mixing bowl. Stir together everything else, dump it over the cabbage, and toss to coat. Great right away, even better with a few hours of chilling.

5 servings, each with 75 calories, 4 g fat, 2 g protein, 7 g carbohydrate, 2 g fiber

Note: *Alternatively, stir up the mayo and yogurt with a good dollop of the sauce on the next page.*

Balsamic-Mustard Sauce

I didn't know where else to put this recipe, but it was too good to leave out. The inspiration for this was a recipe for a clone of an old southern favorite called Durkee Famous Sauce. Being an unregenerate Yankee (New Jersey roots back to before the Revolution), I haven't tried Durkee Famous Sauce—haven't even seen it in the grocery store—but I'd heard about it. It's famous, after all. I'd long been curious about it.

So I adapted the recipe, substituting for the sugar and flour and using balsamic vinegar and spicy brown mustard for extra flavor. I have no idea how this compares to the original, but it's truly terrific in its own right. A dollop will add an extra kick to anything from coleslaw to cocktail sauce.

The recipe makes quite a lot. Mine kept for a good six weeks in a snap-top container in the fridge.

½ cup water
1½ teaspoons guar
½ cup balsamic vinegar
2 tablespoons balsamic vinegar
1 tablespoon salt
½ cup Splenda
1 egg
¼ cup spicy brown mustard
4 tablespoons butter, in pieces

Put everything but the butter in your blender and blend till smooth and thick. Pour/scrape into a saucepan over very low heat.

Warm your sauce *slowly*, stirring constantly. When it's hot, whisk in the butter a bit at a time, letting each addition melt and become amalgamated before adding more. When all the butter is blended in, let your sauce cook for another few minutes, then pour into a snap-top container and refrigerate.

32 servings of about 1½ tablespoons, each with 19 calories, 2 g fat, trace protein, 1 g carbohydrate

Lunch-with-Virginia Salad

I made this for a girls'-lunch-with-wine with my pal Virginia Hudson, and we both loved it. We also agreed that while this is wonderful as a side salad, adding protein would turn it into a terrific main dish. Diced cooked chicken or turkey would be good, as would salad shrimp, flaked crabmeat, or even diced leftover steak or roast beef. Take your pick.

> ½ cup extra-virgin olive oil
> ½ cup peanut oil
> ½ cup white wine vinegar
> ¼ cup grated Parmesan cheese
> 1 tablespoon Splenda or sugar
> 1 teaspoon celery seed
> ½ teaspoon pepper
> ½ teaspoon dry mustard
> ¼ teaspoon paprika
> 1 clove garlic, crushed
> ½ head cauliflower
> ¾ cup cooked wild rice
> 1 6-ounce jar marinated artichoke hearts,
>   drained and chopped
> 1½ cups frozen peas
> ½ green bell pepper, diced
> 5 scallions, including the crisp greens, sliced
> ½ cup drained and chopped oil-packed
>   sun-dried tomatoes
> 1 teaspoon butter
> ¼ cup slivered almonds

Whisk together the first ten ingredients, everything from the extra-virgin olive oil through the garlic. This is your dressing. Set it aside while you assemble your salad.

Trim the leaves and the bottom of the stem from the cauliflower and whack it into chunks. Run the chunks through the shredding disk of your food processor. Dump the shredded cauliflower into a microwavable casserole with a lid. Add a couple of tablespoons of water, cover, and nuke on high for 6 minutes.

While the cauliflower is cooking, get out a big darned salad bowl. Put the wild rice in it. Add your marinated artichoke hearts and your peas—don't bother to thaw them. Throw the diced pepper, scallions, and sun-dried tomatoes into the salad bowl too.

By now your microwave should beep. Pull out your cauliflower, drain it well, and throw it in with the wild rice and other vegetables. Stir everything up. Your cauliflower will thaw your peas, and the frozen peas will cool your cauliflower!

In a small skillet over medium heat, melt your butter. Add the slivered almonds and stir until they're golden. Add them to the salad.

Give your dressing a final whisk, pour it over your salad, and stir it up well. Serve it right away if you like or chill till mealtime. If you let it wait, give it another stir right before serving.

10 servings, each with 309 calories, 26 g fat, 6 g protein, 16 g carbohydrate, 4 g fiber

Note: Look for teeny boxes of wild rice with the other rice in your grocery store. Don't buy "wild and long-grain rice blend." All the grains should be dark brown. Cook according to package directions and stash it in a snap-top container in your freezer. Then you'll have wild rice on hand whenever you want it!

Classic Unpotato Salad

This is a delicious salad, but here's the big picture: I have made at least a dozen different potato salad recipes, substituting cauliflower for the potatoes, and they've all come out great. Please, try your own favorite potato salad recipe with cauliflower!

½ head cauliflower
2 tablespoons wine vinegar
½ teaspoon salt
½ teaspoon pepper
3 hard-boiled eggs, peeled and chopped
1 large rib celery, diced
¼ cup diced bread-and-butter pickles
5 scallions, including the crisp greens, sliced thin
2 tablespoons minced fresh parsley
½ cup light or regular mayonnaise
2 tablespoons brown mustard

Trim the leaves and the very bottom of the stem off your cauliflower. Cut the rest into ½-inch chunks. Put your chunks in a microwavable casserole with a lid, add a couple of tablespoons of water, cover, and nuke on high for 9 minutes.

While your cauliflower is cooking, mix together the vinegar, salt, and pepper in a big mixing bowl.

When your microwave beeps, pull out your cauliflower, uncover it immediately to stop the cooking, drain it, and dump it into the mixing bowl. Stir it up with the seasoned vinegar. Add the eggs, celery, pickles, scallions, and parsley.

Add the mayo and mustard and mix everything up. It's best if you can chill it for an hour or two, but I've been known to eat it straight out of the mixing bowl.

4–5 servings; assuming 5, each will have 139 calories, 8 g fat, 6 g protein, 9 g carbohydrate, 2 g fiber

Easy Pea Salad

This is a retread of a popular salad from the mid–20th century. Back then it was made with canned peas. I think the thawed, uncooked frozen peas are better—fresher tasting, with no mushy texture—but the original version has its charm too. One can of peas, drained, can be substituted for the thawed frozen ones, if you like.

> 1½ cups frozen peas, thawed
> ¼ cup finely diced red onion
> ¼ cup shredded cheddar cheese
> ¼ cup light mayonnaise
> 1 teaspoon Splenda or sugar
> 1 teaspoon spicy brown mustard
> Salt to taste

Quick and easy: throw the peas, onion, and cheese into a mixing bowl. Stir everything else together, dump it on the pea mixture, and stir it up.

3 servings, each with 147 calories, 7 g fat, 6 g protein, 13 g carbohydrate, 4 g fiber

Middle East/Southwest Fusion Salad

Salads of cucumber, tomato, and onion, dressed with olive oil and lemon juice, are common in Middle Eastern cuisine. The avocado, cilantro, and cumin are southwestern. The two together are fresh and wonderful! Perfect with grilled steak or chicken on a hot summer night.

> ¼ cup extra-virgin olive oil
> 2 teaspoons ground cumin
> 1 lemon
> ½ large cucumber, sliced
> 2 medium tomatoes, sliced into thin wedges
> 1 avocado, quartered, peeled, pitted,
>   and sliced crosswise
> ⅛ large red onion, sliced paper-thin
> ¼ cup chopped fresh cilantro
> ½ teaspoon salt

This salad is best served absolutely fresh, so assemble it right before you're planning to serve it—holding it for even a half hour changes it. It's certainly still tasty but not as wonderful.

Mix together the olive oil and cumin and reserve. Squeeze the juice from the lemon into another little dish and set that aside too.

Assemble the veggies and cilantro in a nonreactive mixing bowl. Pour on the olive oil mixture and toss. Pour on the lemon juice and then sprinkle on the salt, toss again, and serve immediately.

6 servings, each with 151 calories, 14 g fat, 1 g protein, 7 g carbohydrate, 2 g fiber

Vietnamese Cucumber Salad

I love cucumber salad in any form. This one is Vietnamese in inspiration, sweet and tart.

> 1 large cucumber, halved and sliced
> 1 large shallot, minced
> ½ jalapeño, seeded and minced
> 1 tablespoon lime juice
> ¼ cup rice vinegar
> 3 tablespoons Splenda or sugar
> ½ teaspoon salt
> 3 tablespoons minced fresh cilantro

In a nonreactive mixing bowl, combine the sliced cucumber with the shallot and jalapeño. Now, go wash your hands well with soap and water! If you don't, you'll be sorry the next time you touch your eyes or nose.

Combine the lime juice, vinegar, Splenda, and salt and pour over the salad. Stir. Add the cilantro and stir again. You can serve this right away, but 15–20 minutes of chilling time lets the flavors blend. Best eaten the same day, though.

4 servings, each with 20 calories, trace fat, 1 g protein, 5 g carbohydrate, 1 g fiber

Fruit Salad with Poppy Seed Dressing

Here's a salad that makes the most of summer's bounty.

> 2 nectarines (you could use peaches, but you'd need to peel them)
> 10 strawberries
> 1 cup blueberries
> 4 teaspoons Splenda or sugar
> 4 teaspoons lemon juice
> 2 tablespoons oil
> 2 pinches dry mustard
> ½ teaspoon poppy seeds
> ⅛ teaspoon salt

Halve your nectarines and remove the pits, then dice—I don't bother to peel first. Put in a pretty glass bowl.

Halve your strawberries lengthwise, then slice and add to the nectarines. Throw your blueberries in.

Now whisk together everything else and pour over the fruit. Toss to coat and stash in the fridge for an hour or so before serving. Or just yum it down right away if you can't wait.

4 servings, each with 128 calories, 8 g fat, 1 g protein, 16 g carbohydrate, 3 g fiber

7

Main-Dish Salads
and Soups

love one-dish meals! I especially love main-dish salads during warm weather and soups in cold weather. Both offer tremendous variety and an unbeatable combination of flavor, texture, variety, and outstanding nutrition. And there aren't as many dishes to wash.

I never tire of trying new salads at home. Please, feel free to invent main-dish salads. They're simple.

One of the easiest bag lunches I know is this: Put several handfuls of bagged salad mix—whatever you like—in a snap-top container. Throw in any protein you have on hand: leftover chicken, turkey, ham, or steak—cut into strips or cubes. If you have no leftovers, use hard-boiled eggs, shredded cheese, or take along a single-serving can or pouch of tuna. Keep packets of dressing in your purse or desk drawer or a bottle of dressing in the break room fridge. (Unpaid plug: I like Newman's Own salad dressings. They use real ingredients, not chemical junk, and they don't use a bunch of corn syrup.) When lunchtime rolls around, pour the dressing on your salad, and devour. Simple, but very satisfying.

But if you'd like to raise the main-dish salad to an art form, here are some ways to do it.

Tomatoes Stuffed with Curried Tuna Salad

This trick of stuffing tomato "flowers" makes any tuna, chicken, egg, or ham salad special (and more nutritious). But when you spark that tuna salad with curry, ginger, currants, and cashews, it becomes really amazing.

> 1 6-ounce can chunk light tuna packed in water
> 1 rib celery, diced
> 3 scallions, including the crisp greens, sliced
> 1 tablespoon dried currants
> 3 tablespoons light mayonnaise
> 1½ teaspoons curry powder
> ½ teaspoon grated fresh ginger
> 2 medium tomatoes
> 2 lettuce leaves for serving
> 2 tablespoons chopped roasted salted cashews

Drain your tuna and dump it into a mixing bowl. Add the celery and scallions to the tuna along with the currants.

Stir together the mayonnaise, curry powder, and ginger. Now add to the tuna and mix to combine.

Cut the cores out of your tomatoes. Cut each into eight wedges, vertically, leaving the skin intact at the bottom. Open up each tomato into a "flower."

Line two serving plates with pretty lettuce leaves and place a tomato on each.

At the last minute, stir your chopped cashews into the tuna salad. Then divide the mixture between the tomatoes and serve.

2 servings, each with 255 calories, 10 g fat, 25 g protein, 17 g carbohydrate, 3 g fiber

Colorful Dill Egg Salad

You'll thank me for this recipe the week after Easter! I like to wrap this salad in lettuce leaves, but it would be truly gorgeous stuffed into a tomato.

6 hard-boiled eggs, peeled and chopped
2 large ribs celery, diced
½ red bell pepper, diced
6 scallions, including the crisp greens, sliced
¼ cup ranch dressing
¼ cup light mayonnaise
½ teaspoon lemon pepper
1 teaspoon dried dill

Put the chopped eggs into a mixing bowl. Add the celery, pepper, and scallions.

Mix together everything else and pour it over the salad. Stir it up and serve.

3 servings, each with 325 calories, 25 g fat, 15 g protein, 9 g carbohydrate, 2 g fiber

Chicken–Smoked Gouda Salad

A great flavor combination. Feel free to use bagged mixed greens instead of the romaine and red leaf.

> 8 ounces boneless, skinless chicken breast
> Salt and pepper to taste
> 1 teaspoon olive oil
> 2 slices bacon
> 4 cups torn romaine lettuce
> 4 cups torn red leaf lettuce
> ¼ cup shredded smoked Gouda cheese
> ¼ cup very thinly sliced red onion
> Apricot-Mustard Dressing (recipe follows)

Put your chicken in a resealable plastic bag and use the nearest heavy, blunt object to pound it out to an even ½-inch thickness. Salt and pepper it lightly, then start it sautéing in the olive oil. You'll want to give it 4 minutes per side and cook till golden and cooked through but not dried out. (Or you could cook it in your electric tabletop grill.)

Cook your bacon—I'd put mine on my microwave bacon rack or in a glass pie plate and nuke it for 2 minutes on high.

Put your greens, Gouda, and onion in a big salad bowl. Pour on the dressing, and toss till every leaf is coated. Pile the salad on two plates.

When your chicken is done, slice or cube it and top your salads with it. Crumble a slice of bacon over each and serve.

2 servings, each with 375 calories, 21 g fat, 34 g protein, 12 g carbohydrate, 4 g fiber

Apricot-Mustard Dressing

I'm putting this dressing by itself because I want you to think of it not just as a salad dressing but also when you need a dipping sauce for chicken, pork, or seafood.

> 1 tablespoon low-sugar apricot preserves
> 1 tablespoon apple cider vinegar
> 1 tablespoon olive oil
> 1 tablespoon light mayonnaise
> 1 teaspoon Dijon or spicy brown mustard
> 1 teaspoon Splenda or sugar
> Scant ⅛ teaspoon pepper
> Pinch salt or Vege-Sal

Just mix everything together. That's it!

Enough for 2–3 servings of salad, the whole batch with 185 calories, 17 g fat, trace protein, 8 g carbohydrate, trace fiber

Chicken Slaw with Honey-Mustard Dressing

Throw in an extra piece or two when you're roasting chicken, buy a sack of preshredded coleslaw, and this is a snap. Feel free to make this with leftover turkey too.

>   1 cup diced cooked chicken
>   2 cups shredded cabbage
>   2 scallions, including the crisp greens, sliced thin
>   ½ teaspoon butter
>   2 tablespoons slivered almonds
>   3 tablespoons light mayonnaise
>   (or regular, if you prefer)
>   2 teaspoons spicy brown or Dijon mustard
>   2 teaspoons honey or Splenda
>   1 teaspoon balsamic vinegar
>   Salt and pepper to taste

In a mixing bowl, combine the diced chicken, shredded cabbage, and sliced scallions.

Melt the butter in a skillet and stir over medium heat and toast the almonds until they're golden. Throw them in the mixing bowl too.

In a small dish, stir together the mayonnaise, mustard, honey or Splenda, and vinegar. Pour over the salad and toss to coat. Salt and pepper to taste and serve.

2 servings, each with 275 calories, 13 g fat, 25 g protein, 14 g carbohydrate, 3 g fiber

Grilled Chicken Salad with Spinach and Apples

A few simple ingredients add up to a salad that's truly delicious—and overwhelmingly nutritious.

> 8 ounces boneless, skinless chicken breast
> Salt and pepper to taste
> 3 tablespoons olive oil
> 3 tablespoons apple cider vinegar
> 2 teaspoons Splenda or sugar
> 1 small garlic clove, peeled and crushed
> 6 cups bagged baby spinach
> 1 small apple, cored and diced
> 2 scallions, including the crisp greens, sliced
> ¼ cup shredded Romano or Parmesan cheese

Cut your chicken into two 4-ounce portions. I put mine in a resealable plastic bag and pound it lightly to an even thickness, about ½ inch, but you can skip this if you want. Either way, salt and pepper both sides, then either throw the chicken into a hot skillet coated with a little nonstick cooking spray (or olive oil) or toss it onto your electric tabletop grill. You'll want to cook it for 4–5 minutes per side, until golden and cooked through but not dried out.

Put your olive oil, vinegar, Splenda, and garlic into a bowl and whisk together well.

Dump your spinach into a salad bowl and pour on your dressing. Toss well, then pile the spinach onto two plates.

Top each serving with half the diced apple and half the sliced scallion.

When your chicken is done, slice or cube it. Top each salad with half the chicken. Scatter 2 tablespoons of the cheese over each salad and serve.

2 servings, each with 440 calories, 28 g fat, 33 g protein, 18 g carbohydrate, 5 g fiber

Oriental Chicken Salad

This is the sort of thing that you'd pay $12.95 for in a restaurant. Yet despite the intimidating list of ingredients, it's quite simple.

> 8 ounces boneless, skinless chicken breast
> Salt and pepper to taste
> 1 teaspoon olive oil
> 1 teaspoon butter
> 2 tablespoons sliced almonds
> 3 tablespoons Splenda or sugar
> 2 tablespoons rice wine vinegar
> ¼ cup light or regular mayonnaise
> 1 teaspoon spicy brown or Dijon mustard
> ⅛ teaspoon dark sesame oil
> ⅛ teaspoon chili garlic paste
> ⅛ teaspoon soy sauce
> 3 cups chopped romaine lettuce
> 1 cup shredded red cabbage
> 1 cup shredded napa cabbage
> 1 cup fresh mung bean sprouts
> ½ carrot, shredded
> 2 scallions, including the crisp greens, sliced

Put your chicken breast in a resealable plastic bag and use any handy heavy object to pound it to an even ½-inch thickness. Salt and pepper both sides lightly. Add the oil to a skillet over medium-high heat and add the chicken breast. You want to give it 4–5 minutes per side, till it's golden and done through but not dried out. (Alternatively, you can use your electric tabletop grill to do this step.)

In your smallest skillet, melt the butter over medium-low heat and add the sliced almonds.

While the chicken and almonds are cooking, make your dressing. Measure the Splenda or sugar, vinegar, mayo, mustard, sesame oil, chili garlic paste, and soy sauce into a small bowl and whisk till smooth. Now stir your almonds—you don't want to burn them; just brown them a little.

Assemble all the veggies in a big darned salad bowl. Pour on the dressing and toss vigorously till everything is coated evenly. Pile the salad on two plates.

Throw your cooked chicken onto your chopping board, slice or cube it, and divide it between the two salads. Top each with a tablespoon of almonds and serve.

2 servings, each with 368 calories, 19 g fat, 32 g protein, 19 g carbohydrate, 5 g fiber

Quasi-Asian Citrus Chicken Salad

I've been known to eat this straight out of the mixing bowl. Yum!

1½ teaspoons butter
¼ cup slivered almonds
1 cup diced cooked chicken
½ cup diced celery
½ cup sliced canned water chestnuts, each slice halved
¼ cup sliced scallions, including the crisp greens
¼ cup light or regular mayonnaise
1 tablespoon lime juice
2 drops orange extract
1½ teaspoons soy sauce
1½ teaspoons Splenda or sugar
¼ teaspoon grated fresh ginger
¼ teaspoon chili garlic paste

In a small skillet over medium heat, melt the butter and start browning the almonds.

Meanwhile, put the chicken, celery, water chestnuts, and scallions into a mixing bowl. Stir your almonds! When they're golden, remove them from the heat.

Mix together the mayo, lime juice, orange extract, soy sauce, Splenda or sugar, ginger, and chili garlic paste. Pour it over the chicken and veggies and stir to coat. Stir in the toasted almonds and serve.

2 servings, each with 478 calories, 35 g fat, 26 g protein, 13 g carbohydrate, 3 g fiber

Walnut-Chicken Salad

This was originally a couscous salad, but the cauliflower is terrific. I know the recipe looks complicated, but it took me about 20 minutes to put together.

> ½ head cauliflower
> 1 tablespoon minced red onion
> 1 clove garlic, peeled and crushed
> 1½ tablespoons rice wine vinegar
> 2 tablespoons olive oil
> 1 teaspoon Splenda or sugar
> ½ teaspoon grated fresh ginger
> ½ teaspoon lemon juice
> 1 teaspoon soy sauce
> 8 ounces boneless, skinless chicken breast
> Salt and pepper to taste
> 2 teaspoons butter
> ½ cup shredded carrot
> 1 bunch scallions, including the crisp greens, sliced
> ¼ cup chopped walnuts
> 6 cups fresh baby spinach

First, the cauliflower—trim the leaves and the very bottom of the stem off the cauliflower and whack it into chunks. Run it through the shredding disk of your food processor. Dump the "rice" into a microwavable casserole with a lid, add a tablespoon or two of water, cover, and nuke it on high for 6 minutes.

Now make your dressing: Put your onion and garlic in a small bowl. Add the vinegar, olive oil, Splenda, ginger, lemon juice, and soy sauce. Whisk everything together.

Put your chicken breast in a resealable plastic bag and use a heavy blunt object to pound it out ½ inch thick all over. Salt and pepper lightly on both sides. Spray a medium skillet with nonstick cooking spray, put it over medium heat, and add a teaspoon of the butter. When the skillet's hot, throw in your chicken breast—it'll take 4–5 minutes per side.

Meanwhile, throw your carrot and scallions into a big salad bowl.

Microwave has beeped? Pull out the cauliflower and uncover it right away to stop the cooking.

When your chicken is done, throw it on your chopping board. Melt the other teaspoon of butter and toss your walnuts into the skillet. Stir them in the butter till they smell toasty, then remove from the heat.

OK, time to assemble your salad! Drain your "rice" and dump it into the salad bowl. Give your dressing another stir, pour it over the cauliflower mixture, and toss everything together. Salt and pepper a little if you think it needs it. Now stir in the walnuts.

Pile the baby spinach on two plates. Spoon the cauliflower mixture on top. Slice your chicken breast and divide the chicken between the two servings.

2 servings, each with 459 calories, 30 g fat, 35 g protein, 18 g carbohydrate, 8 g fiber

Chicken-Asparagus Salad

This takes about 15 minutes to put together, but you can stream-line it further by using bottled Dijon vinaigrette.

> 12 ounces boneless, skinless chicken breast
> 1 tablespoon Dijon or spicy brown mustard
> 3 tablespoons plus 2 teaspoons olive oil
> 1 pound asparagus
> 2 tablespoons white wine vinegar
> ¼ teaspoon salt
> ¼ teaspoon pepper
> 1 10-ounce bag Mediterranean blend salad greens
> 1 bunch scallions, sliced
> 2 tablespoons shredded Romano or Parmesan cheese

First, put your chicken breast in a resealable plastic bag and use the nearest heavy blunt object to pound it out to an even ½-inch thickness.

Spray your big skillet with nonstick cooking spray and put it over medium heat.

Spread 1 teaspoon of the mustard evenly over one side of the chicken breast.

Put 2 teaspoons of the olive oil in the skillet and throw in the chicken, mustard side down. Spread the top with another teaspoon of mustard. (Why not just flip the chicken and spread both sides before putting it in the skillet? Because you'll leave a bunch of your mustard on the cutting board; that's why.) You're giving it about 5 minutes per side.

Snap the ends off the asparagus where it wants to break natu-rally. Lay it on your cutting board and cut it into 1-inch lengths. Put it in a microwavable casserole with a lid, add a tablespoon or two of water, cover, and microwave on high for 3 minutes.

Put the rest of the mustard, the remaining 3 tablespoons olive oil, the vinegar, and salt and pepper in a bowl or shaker and mix or shake well.

Dump your bagged greens into a big salad bowl. Pour on your dressing and toss like mad. Pile it onto two big plates. Divide the asparagus between the two salads.

When your chicken is cooked, slice or cube it. Pile that on top of the asparagus.

Scatter the scallions and Romano over the whole thing and serve while the asparagus and chicken are still warm.

2 servings, each with 523 calories, 32 g fat, 47 g protein, 15 g carbohydrate, 7 g fiber

Ham and Pineapple Slaw

Once you bake a ham, you spend the next week figuring out how to use it up. This recipe makes that same old ham fresh again in a way starchy sandwiches and casseroles never could.

> 3 cups shredded napa cabbage
> ½ cup shredded red cabbage
> ½ cup pineapple in ¼-inch dice
> 2 scallions, including the crisp greens, sliced
> 6 ounces cooked ham, cut into ½-inch cubes
> 2 tablespoons rice vinegar
> 2 tablespoons light or regular mayonnaise
> 1 tablespoon spicy brown mustard
> 1 tablespoon Splenda
> ½ teaspoon soy sauce
> ⅛ teaspoon chili garlic paste
> ¼ clove garlic, peeled and crushed
> 1 tablespoon sesame seeds

Throw everything from the cabbage through the ham cubes into a big salad or mixing bowl.

In a small dish, whisk together the rice vinegar, mayo, mustard, Splenda, soy sauce, chili garlic paste, and garlic.

Put your sesame seeds in a small, dry skillet and shake 'em over medium heat for a few minutes, till they smell toasty. (If you're using hulled sesame seeds—the only kind you'll find at your grocery store—they may well pop and jump a bit in the skillet, and they'll turn golden. If you use unhulled sesame seeds from the health food store—my choice, for the higher mineral content—they won't be so dramatic. Just give 'em a few minutes and they'll be fine.)

Now pour the dressing over the salad and toss till everything's coated. Throw in the sesame seeds, toss again, and serve.

2 servings, each with 284 calories, 15 g fat, 19 g protein, 20 g carbohydrate, 4 g fiber

Note: Buy precut chunks of fresh pineapple in the produce department and just dice 'em up further.

Soups

Soup is wonderful stuff, true comfort food. But if you read the labels on the soup cans in your grocery store, you'll discover that most of them are loaded with starch. Rice, noodles, potatoes, legumes, or cornstarch thickeners—it's hard to find a soup that doesn't have at least one starchy ingredient.

Luckily, soup is easy to make. You'll be dazzled by how much better it is than canned, frozen, or especially (ugh) dried. You know how much better Mom's homemade chocolate chip cookies are than the bagged ones? That's how much better homemade soup is than canned.

If your weeknights are busy, make a double or triple batch of soup over the weekend. Then you can just ladle some into a bowl, zap it in the microwave, and supper's ready!

About Broth

Most soups begin with broth, and the better your broth, the better your soup will be. It is worthwhile to try several brands of packaged broth to find the one you like the best—I think Kitchen Basics brand is good, and it's made from reassuringly real ingredients.

Better yet, make your own broth. It's so easy it's ridiculous. Here's how to always have homemade broth on hand:

Save all your chicken bones in a plastic grocery sack in the freezer. You can save steak bones in another sack, to make beef broth. It doesn't matter if all the meat is gone; stark naked bones will make great broth.

When you have a sackful of bones, dump them into your biggest nonreactive kettle. Cover them with water, add a teaspoon or two of salt and about ¼ cup of vinegar—any kind. Stick it on a back burner, set it to low, and let it simmer till the water's cooked down by about a third. Strain it, dump the bones in the trash, and you've got far better broth than any you can buy. If you have more than you can use right away, freeze your broth in snap-top containers. Having a couple of quarts of broth in the freezer is like money in the bank!

Pho

Say "fuh." I'm putting this recipe first because I want you to try it! This beef noodle soup is Vietnamese comfort food, and it's *wonderful*. I'd never had it till I tried making it myself, and heaven knows I'm not Vietnamese. Yet as I ate this I felt like a kindly grandma was patting me on the head. Sheer bliss.

> 6 cups beef broth, the best you can get
> 1 3-inch cinnamon stick
> 2 whole star anise
> ½ inch fresh ginger, sliced thin
> 10 ounces beef sirloin, well trimmed
> 14 ounces traditional shirataki noodles
> 1 teaspoon chili garlic paste, or to taste
> ¼ cup fish sauce (nuoc mam or nam pla)
> 1 cup mung bean sprouts
> 4 scallions, including the crisp greens, sliced thin
> ¼ cup chopped fresh cilantro
> ¼ cup chopped fresh basil
> 1 lime, cut into wedges

Dump your broth into a kettle or large saucepan and put it over high heat. Add the cinnamon, star anise, and ginger. Bring the broth to a simmer and turn the heat down so the liquid keeps simmering while you do the rest.

Trim any fat off your beef and slice it as thinly as possible, across the grain. (It's easier to thinly slice meat if it's partly frozen.)

Put your shirataki into a strainer and rinse well. Use kitchen shears to snip across them several times in different directions.

When your broth has been simmering for 15 minutes, you can, if you like, skim out the spices with a slotted spoon, but it's not strictly necessary. Now add the beef and stir to keep the slices from sticking together. Add the shirataki and stir in the chili garlic paste and fish sauce. Let the whole thing continue simmering for 5 minutes or so, till the beef's cooked through.

Add the bean sprouts and cook for another minute or so. Then ladle into bowls, top each bowl with scallions, cilantro, and basil, and serve with a wedge of lime to squeeze into it.

3 servings, each with 423 calories, 18 g fat, 42 g protein, 24 g carbohydrate, 6 g fiber

Note: Star anise is available at Asian markets and often in the international food aisle of big grocery stores. It comes whole, not ground, and it really is shaped like a star. Store star anise in a jar with a tight lid.

Creamy Chicken and Artichoke Soup

Simple and quick and elegant. I cloned this from a soup I loved at the Scholar's Inn in Indianapolis, only my version has more chicken.

> 2 teaspoons butter
> ½ small onion, diced small
> 1 quart chicken broth
> 8 ounces boneless, skinless chicken thighs (use breasts instead, if that's what you have on hand, but I like the thigh meat better here)
> 1 14-ounce can artichoke hearts, drained
> 2 tablespoons dry white wine
> ½ cup heavy cream

Over medium-low heat, melt the butter in a big saucepan. Throw in the onion and sauté till it's translucent.

Add the chicken broth, turn up the heat to medium, and bring to a simmer.

Meanwhile, cube your chicken (this is easier if your chicken is half-frozen) and chop your artichoke hearts. Throw them and the chicken into the broth and stir to keep the chicken from sticking together in a clump.

Add the wine. Let the whole thing simmer for another 15–20 minutes.

Stir in the cream and taste. Salt, if it needs it, and serve.

3 servings, each with 318 calories, 23 g fat, 19 g protein, 7 g carbohydrate, 2 g fiber

Curried Coconut Cream of Chicken Soup

So simple and so good! If you don't have coconut milk in the house, cream will do. But why not keep coconut milk in the house?

> 6 cups chicken broth
> 12 ounces boneless, skinless chicken breast
> 3 tablespoons curry powder
> 2 teaspoons chicken bouillon concentrate
> ½ tablespoon butter
> ⅓ cup sliced almonds
> 1 13½-ounce can coconut milk
> Guar or xanthan (optional)

Put your broth in a big saucepan over medium-high heat and let it start warming as you dice the chicken breast. Stir the chicken bouillon into the broth. (If you just dump it in, it will sit in the bottom of the pan and congeal back into a big lump.) Stir in the curry powder and bouillon concentrate and keep it cooking.

In a small skillet, melt your butter over medium heat. Add the almonds and stir them in the butter until they're a nice golden color. Remove from the heat.

Stir the coconut milk into the soup. Let the whole thing cook for another minute or two. Thicken it a bit with your guar or xanthan shaker if you like.

Serve with the toasted almonds on top.

5 servings, each with 394 calories, 30 g fat, 25 g protein, 10 g carbohydrate, 4 g fiber

Easy Chicken Gumbo

When I found frozen gumbo mix in my grocery store, this became inevitable. Feel free to use shrimp instead, or half shrimp, half chicken, or even andouille sausage.

2 slices bacon, diced
1 pound frozen gumbo mix vegetables
2 quarts chicken broth
1 pound boneless, skinless chicken breast,
   thighs, or both
1 14½-ounce can diced tomatoes
2 teaspoons Tabasco sauce, or to taste
1 clove garlic, peeled and crushed
½ teaspoon dried thyme
½ teaspoon pepper
¼ teaspoon cayenne, or to taste

Put your soup kettle or a good big saucepan over medium heat. Put your bacon in the kettle and start it browning.

When the bacon is just starting to get crisp, add the frozen gumbo mix—no need to thaw it first—and the chicken broth.

Cut up your chicken into ½-inch cubes and stir it into the soup (don't just dump it in or it will sink to the bottom of the pot and cook together into a big lump). Stir in everything else, bring the whole thing to a simmer, and let it cook until the veggies are tender. That's it!

5 servings, each with 252 calories, 6 g fat, 31 g protein, 16 g carbohydrate, 2 g fiber

Grandma's Chicken Soup

Of all the grains, barley has the lowest glycemic index, just 22. It's still starchy as heck, of course, so you can't eat bowls and bowls of it. But in a soup like this it's fine—and tastes great.

    2 quarts chicken broth
    ¼ cup barley
    1 large carrot, sliced
    1 medium onion, diced
    1 large rib celery, diced
    1 teaspoon poultry seasoning
    2 bay leaves
    12 ounces boneless, skinless chicken thighs, diced

Put your soup kettle or biggest saucepan over medium heat and dump in the chicken broth. Add the barley and get the whole thing heating.

Meanwhile, cut up your veggies. Throw 'em into the soup along with the poultry seasoning and bay leaves.

Cut your chicken into ½-inch cubes and stir it into the soup. (Don't just dump it in! It'll cook together into a big lump in the bottom of the pot. Stir it in.)

Now you just let the whole thing simmer till the barley's cooked—maybe 40 minutes.

6 servings, each with 227 calories, 12 g fat, 17 g protein, 10 g carbohydrate, 2 g fiber

Note: *You could substitute a package of fettuccine-width tofu shirataki for the barley, for chicken noodle soup.*

Oyster Bisque

Elegant and rich.

> 2 tablespoons butter
> 1 cup finely chopped celery
> 1 cup finely chopped onion
> 1 1-pound tub shucked raw oysters
> Bottled clam juice if needed
> 1 pinch saffron threads
> ¼ teaspoon guar or xanthan
> ¾ teaspoon ground coriander
> ½ teaspoon salt, or to taste
> ⅛ teaspoon cayenne
> 3 cups milk or half-and-half
> ¼ cup chopped fresh parsley

In a large saucepan over medium-low heat, melt your butter and start sautéing the celery and onion. Stir frequently; you want them to soften, not brown.

Meanwhile, put a strainer over a bowl and drain your oysters. Pour the liquid that drains off the oysters into a measuring cup. You want 1 cup. My oysters turned out to have exactly that much liquid on them—go figure! But if you're a little short, make up the difference with bottled clam juice. If you have a little extra oyster liquid, just go ahead and use it. No big deal. For the moment, pop your oysters back into the fridge. You know how seafood is.

When the onion is translucent and the celery softening, add the oyster liquid and the saffron. Bring to a simmer, cover, and cook for 20–30 minutes.

By now your onion and celery should be pretty soft. Your next step depends on what equipment you have. Your aim is to puree the onion and celery. If you have a stick blender, you can puree your vegetables right in the pan. If you don't, you'll have to transfer the mixture to your blender or food processor (with the S-blade in place). Whichever device you use, add the guar or xanthan, coriander, salt, and cayenne and puree them into the celery-onion mixture. Add the milk and puree again. Return to the pan (assuming you took it out in the first place). Turn the heat to low.

Heat slowly—milk scorches easily. While it's heating, pull the oysters out of the fridge and coarsely chop them.

When your soup is simmering, stir in the oysters and parsley. Let it simmer for another 3–5 minutes, till the oysters are cooked through, and serve.

4 servings, each with 264 calories, 15 g fat, 15 g protein, 18 g carbohydrate, 1 g fiber

Seriously Simple Southwestern Sausage Soup

The name says it all! Feel free to use turkey sausage if you prefer.

1 pound bulk pork sausage
1 tablespoon ground cumin
1 teaspoon dried oregano
6 cups chicken broth
1 16-ounce jar salsa
1 can black soybeans

In a kettle or big saucepan, brown and crumble your sausage. When it's done through, drain off any grease.

Now add everything else, bring to a simmer, and serve.

5 servings, each with 456 calories, 39 g fat, 18 g protein, 8 g carbohydrate, 2 g fiber

Super-Chunky Slow-Cooker Vegetable-Beef Soup

This really is super-chunky—more meat and vegetables than broth. If you have a really big slow-cooker, you could double the broth in this recipe and still have a good, chunky soup.

> **1 quart beef broth**
> **1 medium turnip, diced**
> **1 medium carrot, sliced**
> **1 medium onion, diced**
> **1 cup frozen crosscut green beans**
> **1 cup frozen peas**
> **1 15-ounce can diced tomatoes**
> **1 pound boneless beef chuck, well trimmed and**
>   **cut into ½-inch cubes**
> **1 medium rib celery, diced and leaves chopped**
> **2 bay leaves**
> **Salt and pepper to taste**

Just dump the broth into your slow-cooker, cut stuff up, and dump everything except the salt and pepper in too, with the root vegetables—turnip, carrot, and onion—at the bottom. Cover and cook on low for 8–10 hours. Salt and pepper to taste and serve.

5 servings, each with 311 calories, 15 g fat, 26 g protein, 19 g carbohydrate, 3 g fiber

8

Poultry

Do you love chicken? I never tire of the stuff. Chicken is great simply roasted, and it also lends itself to endless variation. It's reliably cheap. The boneless, skinless stuff is even quick to cook.

Too, chicken is a crowd-pleaser. Kids like it, most diets allow it, and it doesn't run afoul (a fowl? sorry) of most religious dietary laws. Truly, it's hard to go wrong with chicken—especially when you have a bunch of great ways to cook it!

I've also included a recipe for using up leftover turkey and one for adding family-pleasing flavor to the cheap-but-bland ground turkey.

To the recipes!

Simple Roasted Chicken

When I was growing up, my mom made roasted chicken at least one night a week. It was easy, it was cheap, and we all liked it. Nothing's changed! Try it with the zippy Cranberry Salsa that follows.

You can roast any cut-up chicken (skin on, bone in) this way. Always roast extra. Then you'll have cold chicken in the fridge for chicken salad or just to eat.

Turn your oven to 375°F or 400°F. Sprinkle your chicken with a little something to season it—you can use:

Good ol' salt and pepper
Barbecue rub
Cajun seasoning
Creole seasoning
Jerk seasoning

If you think about it ahead of time, put your chicken in a resealable plastic bag and pour in enough bottled vinaigrette dressing to coat it. Seal the bag, pressing out the air as you go, turn it to coat the chicken, then throw the bag into the fridge. When it's time to cook, just pour off the dressing and roast.

Or you can pull back the skin and put a few fresh herbs underneath it—sage, oregano, thyme, and marjoram are all good.

However you season your chicken, arrange it in a roasting pan. Slide it into the oven and let it roast for 45 minutes at 400°F or about an hour at 375°F. Baste it once or twice during that time with the drippings in the bottom of the pan. When it's brown and crisp all over, it's done. That's it!

Cranberry Salsa

Not a chicken recipe, but a great way to liven up simple grilled or roasted chicken.

1 jalapeño pepper—2 if you like it really hot!
½ large orange
½ medium red onion
12 ounces fresh cranberries
¾ cup Splenda or sugar, or to taste
3 tablespoons lime juice
¼ teaspoon salt
¼ teaspoon ground cinnamon
½ cup chopped fresh cilantro

Split your jalapeño down the middle and remove the seeds, ribs, and stem. Put in your food processor with the S-blade in place and go wash your hands really well with soapy water before you continue.

Grate the zest of your orange and reserve. Then peel, seed, and put the flesh of the orange in the processor with the jalapeño. Add the onion, cut into a few chunks.

Pulse the food processor till everything is chopped to a medium consistency.

Add the cranberries and pulse till they're chopped to a medium consistency. Transfer the mixture to a nonreactive bowl—glass, plastic, stainless steel, or enamel.

Stir in everything else. Chill for an hour or two to let the flavors marry, then serve with any poultry—or with pork for that matter.

8 servings, each with 40 calories, trace fat, trace protein, 10 g carbohydrate, 2 g fiber

Note: Cranberries are one of the few fruits that are still strictly seasonal; they're available only in the autumn and winter. But they freeze beautifully. Just buy a few extra bags and throw them in your freezer, and you can make cranberry salsa year-round.

Ginger-Sesame Glazed Chicken

This roasted chicken has a great Asian glaze.

>   1 tablespoon grated fresh ginger
>   ½ cup soy sauce
>   ¼ cup lime juice
>   1 tablespoon minced garlic
>   1 tablespoon dark sesame oil
>   1 tablespoon honey
>   2 tablespoons Splenda
>   3 pounds chicken pieces

Mix together everything but the chicken. Place the chicken in a big resealable plastic bag or a nonreactive dish and pour the ginger-soy mixture over it. If using a bag, press the air out and seal, then turn over to coat the chicken. If using a nonreactive dish, turn the chicken over a couple of times to coat. Either way, refrigerate your chicken and let it marinate for at least an hour or two. If marinating in a dish, turn it over at least once during the marinating time.

Preheat your oven to 375°F. Pour the marinade off the chicken into a bowl and reserve.

Lay your chicken skin side up in a roasting pan. Roast for 75 minutes, basting with the reserved marinade every 15–20 minutes; do not baste for at least the final 10 minutes of cooking time.

5 servings, each with 462 calories, 31 g fat, 36 g protein, 9 g carbohydrate, trace fiber

Lemon-Lime Chicken

The tangy marinade enhances the flavor of the chicken itself.

> **3 pounds cut-up chicken, light meat or dark or any combination**
> ¼ **cup lemon juice**
> ¼ **cup lime juice**
> ¼ **cup dry white wine**
> ¼ **cup olive oil**
> **2 cloves garlic, peeled and crushed**
> **1 teaspoon salt or Vege-Sal**
> ⅛ **teaspoon pepper**
> **1 teaspoon Tabasco sauce**
> ¼ **teaspoon dried thyme**

Put your chicken in a big resealable plastic bag or a bowl. Mix together everything else and pour it into the bag. Seal the bag, pressing out the air as you go. Toss the bag into the fridge and let the whole thing marinate for at least a few hours; all day is great. (If you think of it, flip the bag over whenever you stick your head in the fridge, but it's not essential.)

When cooking time comes, preheat your oven to 400°F. Retrieve your bag from the fridge and pour off the marinade into a bowl. Arrange the chicken in a roasting pan.

Roast for about 45 minutes, basting a few times with the reserved marinade. When your chicken is well browned and the juices run clear when you pierce the chicken to the bone, it's done.

6 servings, each with 427 calories, 32 g fat, 29 g protein, 3 g carbohydrate, trace fiber

Cashew-Crusted Chicken

I came up with this while I was making Curried Buttery Cashews (Chapter 5) to send out for Christmas presents. Good as is; even better with the Apricot-Mustard Dressing in Chapter 7 as a dipping sauce.

2½ pounds boneless, skinless chicken breast
1 cup raw cashew pieces
½ teaspoon salt or Vege-Sal
¼ teaspoon garlic powder
¼ teaspoon onion powder
½ teaspoon curry powder
Pinch cayenne
2 tablespoons butter

Pound each chicken breast out to ½ inch thick by putting them in a resealable plastic bag one at a time and whacking with any handy heavy, blunt object. Cut into 6 equal portions.

Put the cashews in your food processor with the S-blade in place, add the seasonings, and pulse till the cashews are chopped medium-fine—you want some texture left. Spread this mixture on a big plate.

One piece at a time, press both sides of each of the pieces of chicken breast in the seasoned cashews.

Spray your biggest skillet with nonstick cooking spray and put it over medium heat. Melt the butter and sauté the chicken about 5 minutes per side, till golden and crisp on the outside and done through. Serve immediately.

6 servings, each with 383 calories, 19 g fat, 46 g protein, 6 g carbohydrate, 1 g fiber

Note: You can use whole raw cashews for this recipe, but at my health food store raw cashew pieces are less than half the price of whole cashews. So that's what I buy.

Chicken Florentine Alfredo

This would make a stunning company dinner, but I've been known to make half the recipe just for my husband and me.

1½ pounds boneless, skinless chicken breast
1½ teaspoons butter
1½ teaspoons olive oil
½ cup chopped mushrooms (I favor cremini and portobello, but the familiar button mushrooms will do fine)
2 cloves garlic
10 ounces frozen chopped spinach, thawed
2 ounces cream cheese
½ cup shredded mozzarella cheese
⅓ cup grated Parmesan cheese
2 tablespoons chopped sun-dried tomatoes
½ teaspoon Italian seasoning
Salt and pepper to taste
½ cup jarred Alfredo sauce

Preheat the oven to 350°F.

One at a time, put your chicken breasts in a big resealable plastic bag and use a heavy, blunt object to pound them out to about ¼-inch thickness. Try to get the pieces roughly the same shape. You'll want four pounded fillets in total. Set aside.

In your big, heavy skillet, warm the butter and olive oil together; then start sautéing the mushrooms. While that's happening, peel and crush your garlic and drain your spinach. Really squeeze it out well—I like to dump it in a strainer and press it with the back of a spoon.

When the mushrooms are soft, stir in the garlic and cook for another minute or two. Then stir in the spinach and let the whole thing get warm.

Now stir in the cream cheese till it's melted. Next, stir in the mozzarella, ¼ cup of the Parmesan, the sun-dried tomatoes, and the Italian seasoning. Salt and pepper to taste.

Spray a baking pan with nonstick cooking spray. Lay two of the pounded chicken breasts in it. Divide the spinach mixture between them and spread it in an even layer, all the way to the edges. Lay the other two pounded breasts on top, making two "sandwiches." Now cut each sandwich into two portions.

Top each sandwich with 2 tablespoons of Alfredo sauce and then with 1½ teaspoons of grated Parmesan.

Bake for 40 minutes. Garnish with a little chopped fresh oregano or basil, if you have some on hand (no big deal if you don't), and serve.

4 servings, each with 440 calories, 24 g fat, 49 g protein, 7 g carbohydrate, 2 g fiber

Orange-Soy-Chicken-Asparagus Stir-Fry

Most stir-fry recipes have a low-glycemic load as long as you don't serve them over rice. The orange makes this one citrusy fresh, yet it isn't enough to spike your blood sugar.

> 1 orange
> 2 tablespoons soy sauce
> ½ clove garlic
> 2 teaspoons Splenda or sugar
> 12 ounces boneless, skinless chicken breast
> ½ pound asparagus
> 1 medium onion, sliced
> 1 tablespoon coconut oil or peanut oil

Grate the zest of your orange and squeeze its juice. In a mixing bowl, combine both with the next three ingredients.

Cube your chicken breast and put it in the bowl with the orange juice mixture. Toss to make sure all the cubes are coated. Let this sit for at least 30 minutes.

Meanwhile, snap the ends off your asparagus where they want to break naturally. Cut it on the diagonal into ½-inch lengths. Peel your onion and cut it into half rounds about ¼ inch thick.

Put a big skillet or wok over highest heat. Fish the chicken out of its marinade with a fork and put it on a plate by the stove, along with the veggies. Reserve the marinade.

When the pan is good and hot, add the oil. When it's hot, throw in the chicken. Stir-fry till all the pink is gone. Scoop the chicken out and put it back in the bowl with the marinade. (Yes, I know the marinade has raw chicken germs in it. Don't panic.)

If the pan needs more oil, add just a touch more. Throw in the asparagus and onion and stir-fry till crisp-tender—the asparagus should be brilliant emerald green.

Dump in the cooked chicken and the marinade and stir it all together. Stir-fry for another few minutes (which will blend flavors and kill those germs) and serve.

2 servings, each with 338 calories, 12 g fat, 41 g protein, 17 g carbohydrate, 4 g fiber

Blue Cheese–Walnut-Pesto Chicken with Noodles

Awfully fancy, considering that you can put it together in 20 minutes flat!

> 16 ounces tofu shirataki, fettuccine style
> ¼ cup chicken broth
> 1 tablespoon butter, divided
> ¼ cup chopped walnuts
> 8 ounces boneless, skinless chicken thighs (or breasts, if you prefer)
> ¼ cup diced onion
> 1 clove garlic, peeled and crushed
> ⅓ cup half-and-half
> 2 tablespoons jarred pesto sauce
> 5½ ounces crumbled blue cheese (I can buy a tub just this size at my grocery)

Open the shirataki and dump it into a strainer. Rinse well. Now put it in a bowl and stir in the chicken broth. Let this sit for about 30 minutes or even all day. (If you want to be able to cook as soon as you get home, do this in a snap-top container or resealable plastic bag and stash in the fridge before you head off to work.)

The rest is quick and easy. Melt a teaspoon of your butter in a small skillet over medium-low heat and stir your walnuts in it until they smell toasty. Remove from the heat and set aside.

Cut your chicken into ½-inch chunks. Melt the rest of your butter in your big, heavy skillet over medium heat and start the chicken and onion sautéing in it.

While that's happening, dump the shirataki and broth into a small saucepan and set over a burner to warm.

When all the pink is gone from your chicken and the onion is translucent, stir in the garlic, half-and-half, and pesto. Now add all but a couple of tablespoons of the blue cheese. Stir until the cheese is melted and the sauce is thick.

Using tongs or a slotted spoon, lift the noodles out of their broth and pile on three plates or bowls. Divide the chicken mixture and sauce between them. Top each with a third of the reserved blue cheese and walnuts and serve.

3 servings, each with 456 calories, 36 g fat, 27 g protein, 6 g carbohydrate, 1 g fiber

Turkey Meat Loaf

Ground turkey is inexpensive, but it's often bland. This turkey meat loaf is bursting with flavor!

> **1 medium carrot**
> **1 medium rib celery**
> **1 medium onion**
> **1 small apple**
> **2 pounds ground turkey**
> **1 tablespoon poultry seasoning**
> **2 tablespoons Worcestershire sauce**
> **2 teaspoons salt or Vege-Sal**
> **½ cup oat bran**
> **1 egg**

Preheat the oven to 350°F.

Using the shredding disk, run the carrot, celery, onion, and apple through your food processor. If yours is like mine, you'll end up with some unshredded produce atop the disk. What the heck—chop that stuff up with a regular old knife or grate it on your box grater and throw it in too.

Dump all your shredded stuff into a big mixing bowl and add everything else. Using clean hands, mush everything together till it's all very well blended.

Pack the mixture into a loaf pan and bake for 45 minutes. Let sit for 10 minutes before serving.

8 servings, each with 216 calories, 10 g fat, 22 g protein, 10 g carbohydrate, 2 g fiber

Creamed Turkey and Vegetables

You'll thank me for this recipe the Saturday after Thanksgiving!

> 1 medium onion, chopped
> 1 tablespoon butter
> 3 cups chicken broth
> 2 cups frozen peas and carrots
> 1 can mushrooms, water and all
> 3 cups diced cooked turkey
> 1½ cups half-and-half
> Guar or xanthan
> Salt and pepper to taste
> 1½ teaspoons poultry seasoning
> 2 packages tofu shirataki noodles, fettuccine style

In a large saucepan, sauté the onion in the butter until translucent.

Add the broth, the peas and carrots, and the mushrooms. Bring to a simmer and cook until the carrots are tender, about 15–30 minutes. (If you prefer, you can speed this up by microwaving your peas and carrots according to the package directions before you add them to the broth.)

Add the turkey and half-and-half. Use your guar or xanthan shaker to thicken to taste—a heavy cream consistency is about right. Salt and pepper and stir in the poultry seasoning. Turn the burner to the lowest heat and keep warm while you . . .

Drain and rinse the shirataki. Stir into the creamed turkey mixture and let simmer another five minutes or so, then serve.

4 servings, each with 391 calories, 22 g fat, 33 g protein, 15 g carbohydrate, 3 g fiber

Smoked Turkey, Sun-Dried Tomato, and Yellow Pepper Pizza

My husband and I had this for New Year's Eve supper. It turned staying home watching video movies into a party! If you don't have a yellow pepper, a green or red one will do; your pizza will still be ultraspecial.

1 yellow bell pepper, sliced thin
½ medium onion, sliced thin
1 clove garlic, peeled and crushed
1 tablespoon olive oil, plus a little for brushing
     the tortillas
¾ pound sliced smoked turkey breast
¾ cup drained oil-packed sun-dried tomatoes
2 tablespoons jarred pesto sauce
2 large low-carb tortillas
1½ cups shredded mozzarella cheese

Preheat the oven to 425°F.

In your big, heavy skillet over medium heat, start sautéing the bell pepper, onion, and garlic in the olive oil.

Cut your slices of smoked turkey breast into 1-inch squares— just cut through all the slices at once. With the S-blade in place, plunk 'em into your food processor. Add the sun-dried tomatoes and the pesto. Pulse till the whole thing is chopped to a medium consistency.

OK, your onions and peppers are a bit softened. Time to assemble pizzas: Lay a large low-carb tortilla on a cookie sheet. Brush it lightly with a little more olive oil. Now spread half the turkey mixture on top. Cover that with half the pepper/onion mixture and top that with ¾ cup shredded mozzarella. Repeat with the second tortilla and the rest of the ingredients.

Bake for about 10 minutes, or until the cheese is melted and getting a few golden spots. Cut into quarters to serve.

4 servings, each with 450 calories, 28 g fat, 34 g protein, 19 g carbohydrate, 9 g fiber

9

Beef

Beef draws a lot of fire. Health-conscious people shun beef or eat it with a sneaking sense of guilt. But it's time to get over your beef phobia.

Beef is darned nutritious stuff. Comparing six ounces of beef flank steak with an equal portion of boneless, skinless chicken breast, the beef has more potassium, iron, thiamine, riboflavin, and folacin and *vastly* more zinc and B_{12}—all for a big 66 extra calories. Both are equally devoid of carbohydrate. Very simply, beef is good for you.

What about beef fat? Isn't it terribly saturated? Half of the fat in beef is unsaturated. Further, half of the saturated fat is in the form of *stearic acid*, a saturated fat that has the same effect on blood fats as olive oil—which is to say, it lowers your bad cholesterol and raises your good cholesterol. Stop worrying.

Better, buy grass-fed beef. Yes, it's pricey, and you'll probably have to go out of your way to find it, but grass-fed beef is on a par with salmon for healthy omega-3 fats. It's also better for the environment.

There's nothing like tucking into a big steak, with a crisp salad on the side and a big glass of red wine, to make you think "What diet?!" So long as you skip the baked potato and "Texas toast," you are now free to think of steak as a healthy dinner.

The same goes for a big pot of chili, a grilled burger, a slab of prime rib—or any of the recipes below!

Burgers

Other countries include ground meat in their cuisines, but America has elevated it to the status of National Dish. I am here to defend the venerable hamburger patty. It's the hamburger's pals that cause the trouble—the bun, the fries, and the soda or shake.

Being a nutrition geek, I did the math. If you eat a quarter-pound burger with cheese, a supersized order of fries, and a giganto-sugared soda, you'll get over 1,600 calories, which—let us face it—is part of the problem right there. But just 450 of those calories come from fat, just 28 percent. Our hypothetical fast-food meal is a perfect illustration of the glycemic-load diet's simple rule—knock out the starch and the sugared beverages and you'll be fine.

So, eat hamburgers! Just eat 'em with a fork, topping a salad, or wrapped in lettuce, rather than on a bun. And skip the fries and the liquid candy. (If you can't resist the fries, stay out of the fast-food joints!)

I like ground chuck best for burgers. It has a great lean-to-fat ratio and a great flavor. When ground chuck goes on sale, I buy twenty pounds or more, make it into six-ounce patties (a little bigger than a third of a pound), and freeze them. Sound like too much work? Look in your grocery store's freezer case. Very likely they have premade hamburger patties, which are a terrific convenience food for us. Just read the label to make sure they have no starchy fillers. (If the burgers are 100 percent beef, the label is likely to boast of it in bold font.)

Whether you make your own or buy premade patties, it's up to you whether you want to pan-broil your burgers, run them under the broiler, or throw them onto your electric tabletop grill. However you cook them, they're quick and easy protein.

But a bunless burger sounds sort of . . . well, plain. You can top it with the usual ketchup, mustard, and pickles if you like. But there are plenty of other things to do to a burger. Try:

A sprinkle of barbecue rub—plus barbecue sauce if you like
Melted mozzarella and pizza sauce
Pepper Jack cheese and salsa
Blue cheese and minced red onion
Sautéed onions, mushrooms, or both
Crumbled feta and chopped olives
Mayonnaise seasoned with crushed garlic and snipped herbs

Of course, you don't have to eat your ground beef in patties—or mixed with Hamburger Helper, which invariably is loaded with noodles, rice, or potatoes. Here are some great ideas to get you going.

Joe

This is how I currently make "Joe's Special," a venerable recipe that apparently started in San Francisco. When my husband and I want a dinner that's fast, easy, filling, and good, this is it. Feel free to play with this; it's hard to make a bad batch of Joe. The immutable basics are ground beef, onion, garlic, spinach, and eggs. But you can use more or less meat, more or fewer eggs. You can leave out the cheese or add more. If you have some mushrooms hanging around the house, they'd be good in here. Some people add a shot of Worcestershire, others a dash or two of Tabasco, still others a little oregano or nutmeg or even coriander. I've even heard of people adding tofu, but that's the sort of thing I prefer not to think about.

> 1½ pounds ground chuck or round
> 1 large onion, chopped
> 3 cloves garlic, peeled and crushed
> 10 ounces frozen chopped spinach, thawed and
>   drained well
> 6 eggs, beaten
> Salt and pepper to taste
> ⅓ cup grated fresh Parmesan cheese

Put your big, heavy skillet over medium heat and throw in your ground chuck or round. Start it browning and crumbling.

When some fat has cooked out of your meat, throw in the onion and garlic. Keep cooking (and crumbling the meat) until all the pink is gone from the meat and the onion is soft and translucent. Tilt the pan, scoop the meat-and-onion mixture to the top of the slope, and use a big spoon to spoon out as much grease as you can.

Now stir in the thawed spinach and the eggs and keep stirring till the eggs are set. Sprinkle the Parmesan over everything and serve.

6 servings, each with 406 calories, 29 g fat, 29 g protein, 5 g carbohydrate, 2 g fiber

Note: Spinach can hold a lot of water! Dump it into a strainer and press it with the back of a spoon. Or, easier, use clean hands and squeeze it hard.

Sloppy Giuseppe

Like Sloppy Joes, only Italian and without the bun. Come to think of it, mushrooms would be good in this, too.

> 1½ pounds ground chuck or round
> 1 large onion, chopped
> 3 cloves garlic, peeled and crushed
> 10 ounces frozen chopped spinach, thawed and
>   drained well
> 1½ cups spaghetti sauce
> 1 teaspoon Italian seasoning
> ⅓ cup grated fresh Parmesan cheese

Put your big, heavy skillet over medium heat and throw in the ground beef. Start it browning and crumbling.

When some grease has cooked out of the meat, throw in your onion and garlic. Keep browning and crumbling till all the pink is gone from the meat and the onion is soft and translucent. Now tilt the skillet and use a spoon to spoon out all the grease you can.

Stir in the spinach, spaghetti sauce, and Italian seasoning. Let the whole thing simmer for 5–10 minutes, then serve with the Parmesan on top.

5 servings, each with 435 calories, 31g fat, 29 g protein, 10 g carbohydrate, 4 g fiber

Jersey Girl Chili

So good! It's the faint Italian accent that gives this chili its New Jersey attitude. And I ought to know; I grew up there.

12 ounces mild Italian sausage
1½ pounds ground chuck
2 medium onions, chopped
2 cloves garlic, peeled and crushed
1 14½-ounce can diced tomatoes
1 8-ounce can tomato sauce
¼ cup dry red wine
2 tablespoons lemon juice
⅓ cup chili powder
3 tablespoons ground cumin
1 tablespoon dried basil
1 tablespoon dried oregano
1½ teaspoons salt or Vege-Sal
1½ teaspoons pepper
1 teaspoon beef bouillon concentrate
¾ cup water
1 15-ounce can black soybeans

Put your biggest skillet over medium heat and throw in the sausage and ground chuck. (If your sausage is in links, remove the casings so you can crumble it with the beef.) Brown and crumble the two together until cooked through. When the meat is done, drain off the fat.

Add the onions and garlic and continue cooking, stirring from time to time, till the onions have softened a little. Then simply add everything else, stirring carefully, since, if your skillet is like mine, it will be very full!

Turn the heat down and simmer for 40–45 minutes. Serve with a dollop of sour cream and a handful of shredded cheddar.

8 servings, each with 441 calories, 33 g fat, 24 g protein, 13 g carbohydrate, 3 g fiber

Someone Else's Mother-in-Law's Meat Loaf

I adapted this from a recipe I found online. The woman who'd posted it said her mother-in-law made the best meat loaf ever and then gave the recipe. It called for a lot of bread crumbs, but I fixed that. Using modest quantities of oat bran works well in meat loaf recipes in general. This is great warmed up the next day too.

> 1 pound ground chuck
> 8 ounces bulk pork sausage
> 1 egg
> ½ cup oat bran
> 1 green bell pepper, diced fine
> 1 large rib celery, chopped fine
> 1 medium carrot, shredded
> 1 medium onion, chopped fine
> 1 8-ounce can tomato sauce
> ¼ teaspoon dry mustard
> ¼ teaspoon dried sage
> ¼ teaspoon dried thyme
> 1 teaspoon salt or Vege-Sal
> ¼ teaspoon pepper
> ⅛ teaspoon ground nutmeg

Preheat the oven to 350°F.

Put the meats, egg, and oat bran in a big mixing bowl. Add the vegetables.

Measure out ½ cup of the tomato sauce and stir the seasonings into it. Then add to the bowl and, using clean hands, squish everything together very well.

Turn into a greased loaf pan and pat out evenly. Top with the remaining tomato sauce.

Bake for 75 minutes. As soon as the meat loaf comes out of the oven, drain off the fat that has accumulated. Then let it sit for 10 minutes before slicing and serving.

6 servings, each with 419 calories, 32 g fat, 21 g protein, 13 g carbohydrate, 3 g fiber

Frenchified Meat Loaf

The recipe I adapted this from called for *herbes de Provence*, which I didn't have on hand. It also called for a lot more bread. So I made it this way, and it was wildly flavorful.

> 1 pound ground chuck
> ½ pound bulk mild pork sausage
> 2 slices low-carb whole-grain bread, in fine crumbs,
>   *or* ⅓ cup oat bran
> ½ cup finely chopped onion
> 1 clove garlic, minced
> ¼ cup chopped fresh parsley
> ¼ cup dry red wine
> 1 egg
> 1 tablespoon Dijon or spicy brown mustard
> ½ teaspoon dried savory
> ½ teaspoon dried thyme
> ¼ teaspoon ground rosemary
> ½ teaspoon salt or 1 teaspoon Vege-Sal
> ¼ teaspoon pepper

Preheat the oven to 350°F.

Dump all your ingredients into a big bowl. Use clean hands to squish it all together until it's really well mixed.

Now pack your meat loaf mixture into a loaf pan and bake for 50–60 minutes. Remove from the oven, drain the fat out of the pan, and let the loaf sit for 5–10 minutes before slicing and serving.

8 servings, each with 304 calories, 24 g fat, 16 g protein, 4 g carbohydrate, 1 g fiber

Steak

It's hard to improve on a perfectly broiled steak. But if you'd like to gild the lily, you could add:

sautéed mushrooms, sautéed onions, or both
a dollop of garlic butter
guacamole, homemade or store-bought

Or one of these easy steak toppers:

Horseradish Sauce

Horseradish and beef are a classic combination.

¼ cup mayonnaise (I use light because it's less likely to "break" when it hits the hot steak)
2 tablespoons sour cream
1 scallion, including the crisp greens, minced fine
1 tablespoon prepared horseradish

Just mix everything together and spoon over steak.

6 servings, each with 35 calories, 3 g fat, trace protein, 1 g carbohydrate, trace fiber

Blue Cheese Pesto Butter

This is the sort of recipe that would make the low-fat faithful blanch. And it's so good!

> **6 tablespoons butter, softened**
> **3 tablespoons crumbled blue cheese**
> **1½ tablespoons jarred pesto sauce**

Just run everything through your food processor. Put a dollop on each serving of hot steak.

6 servings, each with 136 calories, 14 g fat, 2 g protein, trace carbohydrate, trace fiber

Chipotle Butter

A steak topped with this smoky-hot butter, a big green salad with orange segments in it, and a cold light beer. What diet?

> **4 tablespoons butter**
> **1 chipotle chile canned in adobo, plus a teaspoon of the sauce**
> **1 clove garlic, peeled**
> **2 tablespoons chopped onion**
> **1 tablespoon chopped fresh cilantro**

Just run everything through your food processor (using the S-blade) until smooth.

6 servings, each with 70 calories, 8 g fat, trace protein, 1 g carbohydrate, trace fiber

Fire Steak

But only a small fire. This won't burn your taste buds off.

> ¼ cup Tabasco sauce
> 3 tablespoons water
> 1 tablespoon Sucanat *or* 1 tablespoon Splenda and
>   ⅛ teaspoon blackstrap molasses
>   (or the darkest available)
> 1 pound beef rib-eye or a good thick T-bone

Mix together everything but the steak.

Pierce your steak all over with a fork. Put in a resealable plastic bag and pour in the marinade. Seal the bag, pressing out the air as you go. Turn to coat the steak with the marinade. Throw the bag into the fridge and let it sit—all day if you can, but at least for an hour or two.

Now broil or grill close to the heat, until done to your taste, and serve.

3 servings, each with 278 calories, 14 g fat, 31 g protein, 5 g carbohydrate, trace fiber

Note: *To turn an inexpensive chuck pot roast into a great, grillable steak, first make a double batch of this marinade. Then sprinkle your chuck steak with ½ teaspoon of meat tenderizer and pierce the steak all over. Flip and repeat on the other side, including another ½ teaspoon of meat tenderizer. Then marinate and grill as for Fire Steak. You can eat great on a budget!*

Island Steak

These seasonings are classically Caribbean.

½ medium onion
1 jalapeño pepper
¼ cup Splenda or Sucanat
¼ cup lime juice
¼ cup soy sauce
1 tablespoon grated fresh ginger
½ teaspoon ground allspice
½ teaspoon dried thyme
½ teaspoon paprika
3 cloves garlic, peeled
1½ teaspoons meat tenderizer
2 pounds boneless chuck roast, 1½–2 inches thick

Throw everything but the chuck into your food processor with the S-blade in place and pulse until the onion, jalapeño, and garlic are minced quite fine and you have a slurry.

Lay your chuck in a nonreactive dish and pierce it all over with a fork. Flip and pierce the other side too. Pour the marinade over the steak and flip it over again, making sure it's coated thoroughly on both sides. Now stash the whole thing in the fridge for several hours; overnight is even better.

When dinnertime rolls around, pull out your steak and pour off the marinade into a nonreactive pan. Broil the steak close to the flame till it's done to your liking; timing will depend on how thick it is. In the meanwhile, bring the marinade to a boil and boil it hard for a few minutes to kill the raw meat germs. Serve with the steak.

6 servings, each with 337 calories, 24 g fat, 25 g protein, 5 g carbohydrate, 1 g fiber

Beef and Bok Choy

I invented this simple stir-fry when our adorable neighbor Keith brought us some baby bok choy he'd grown. It's so good! Definitely worth going to the grocery store for the bok choy if you're not lucky enough to have green-thumbed neighbors.

> 8 ounces boneless beef chuck
> 3 tablespoons soy sauce
> ½ teaspoon meat tenderizer
> 2 teaspoons dark sesame oil
> 1 clove garlic, minced
> 1 teaspoon honey or Splenda
> ¼ teaspoon chili garlic paste
> 2 tablespoons peanut oil
> 3 cups chopped bok choy (just quarter the heads
>   lengthwise for baby bok choy)

Slice your beef across the grain as thinly as you can. (It helps to have the beef half-frozen when you do this.) In a nonreactive bowl, mix together the soy sauce, meat tenderizer, sesame oil, garlic, honey or Splenda, and chili garlic paste. Add the beef slices and toss to coat with the soy mixture. Let sit for at least 30 minutes.

Put your wok or a big skillet over highest heat. Add the oil and let it get good and hot. Meanwhile, use a fork or tongs to lift the beef out of the marinade. Reserve the marinade.

Throw your drained beef slices into the skillet and stir-fry till the pink is gone. Add the bok choy and stir-fry for another minute or two. Pour the marinade over the stir-fry, stir-fry for another couple of minutes, and serve.

2 servings, each with 437 calories, 36 g fat, 21 g protein, 8 g carbohydrate, 1 g fiber

Balsamic Slow-Cooker Short Ribs

Slow-cooker easy, but company good! Feel free to cut this recipe in half if you like. Personally, I love having leftovers in the fridge for a fast meal. Serve with Fauxtatoes or Cauliflower-Potato Mash (you'll find both recipes in Chapter 6).

> 3 pounds meaty beef short ribs
> 1 onion, sliced thin
> 8 ounces sliced mushrooms
> 1 clove garlic, peeled and crushed
> ¼ cup balsamic vinegar
> ¼ cup apple cider vinegar
> 2 tablespoons Sucanat *or* 2 tablespoons Splenda and
>   ½ teaspoon blackstrap molasses
> 1 tablespoon soy sauce
> ½ teaspoon dry mustard
> 1 tablespoon ketchup
> ½ teaspoon chili powder
> 1½ teaspoons beef bouillon concentrate
> Guar or xanthan

Preheat your broiler.

Arrange the short ribs on your broiler rack and start 'em broiling about 6 inches from the heat. You want to brown them for about 5–7 minutes per side.

Meanwhile, throw your onion, mushrooms, and garlic into the bottom of your slow-cooker.

Mix together everything else but the guar or xanthan.

When the ribs are browned all over, place them on top of the onion and mushrooms. Now pour the sauce over the whole thing. Cover the slow-cooker and set the sucker on low. Let it all cook for 6–8 hours.

When time's almost up, make your Fauxtatoes or Cauliflower-Potato Mash and dish 'em up. Then uncover the slow-cooker and use tongs to pull the ribs out onto the plates, next to the mash.

Use your guar or xanthan shaker to thicken up the sauce left in the pot, then spoon the sauce and veggies over the whole thing and serve.

8 servings, each with 375 calories, 21 g fat, 40 g protein, 5 g carbohydrate, 1 g fiber

Braised Short Ribs

Ribs with tomatoes, wine, and herbs. How much better can it get? I'd probably serve this, like the preceding recipe, with Fauxtatoes or Cauliflower-Potato Mash (see Chapter 6), but it's up to you.

> 2½ pounds meaty beef short ribs
> 2 slices bacon
> 1 medium onion, cut into big chunks
> 2 medium carrots, cut into big chunks
> 2 cloves garlic, peeled and crushed
> 1 14-ounce can diced tomatoes with garlic, basil, and oregano
> ¼ cup dry red wine
> 1 teaspoon beef bouillon concentrate
> 1 teaspoon dried basil
> ½ teaspoon dried rosemary
> ¼ cup chopped fresh parsley

Preheat your broiler and spray your broiler rack with nonstick cooking spray. Arrange the short ribs on the rack. Broil 4 inches or so from the heat, turning now and then, till they're brown and crispy all over.

Meanwhile, give your big, heavy skillet a shot of the same nonstick cooking spray and put it over medium-low heat. Snip your bacon into it with your kitchen shears and start the bits cooking.

Put your onion and carrots into the food processor with the S-blade in place and pulse till everything's chopped to a medium consistency. Dump into the skillet, where some fat should have cooked out of the bacon by now. Sauté till the onions are getting a little brown around the edges. Stir in the crushed garlic, cook for another minute, then dump the whole kit and kaboodle into the bottom of your slow-cooker.

Your short ribs are still browning—don't forget to turn them! Now dump the tomatoes, wine, beef bouillon concentrate, basil, and rosemary into the slow-cooker. Stir till the bouillon concentrate is dissolved.

When your ribs are brown all over, plunk 'em into the middle of the stuff in the slow-cooker. Scatter the parsley over everything, cover, and set to low. Let cook for 6–8 hours.

6 servings, each with 443 calories, 24 g fat, 45 g protein, 8 g carbohydrate, 1 g fiber

10

Pork and Lamb

Pork is nothing if not controversial. It is the world's most popular meat, yet it is also the subject of religious taboos. Many people think of pork as an indulgence, even a guilty pleasure. This is a shame. Pork is indisputably delicious and also highly nutritious. Pork is a protein, of course, but it is also a surprisingly rich source of potassium and a good source of B vitamins. As for the much-maligned pork fat, it actually has more monounsaturates than saturates. Add to this the fact that pork is inexpensive! Enjoy pork guiltlessly as often as you like.

As for lamb, it is my favorite meat. I grew up loving lamb chops and roast leg of lamb, so it was a surprise to learn that many people have never even tried it. I hope you have, and if you haven't, I hope you will.

Before we get into the recipes, one idea so simple I was reluctant to give it full recipe status: I adore pork shoulder steaks, simply pan broiled in a little olive oil and sprinkled with Creole seasoning or barbecue rub. With a big pile of coleslaw on the side, this is one of my favorite meals, and you can put it together in 15 minutes.

Lemon-Mustard Pork Chops

Warm, sunny flavors, and very quick and easy.

> Salt and pepper to taste
> 1½ pounds pork chops
> 2 tablespoons olive oil
> ½ cup chicken broth
> 1½ tablespoons dry vermouth
> 1 teaspoon dried thyme
> 1½ tablespoons Dijon or spicy brown mustard
> 1½ tablespoons lemon juice

Give your big, heavy skillet a shot of nonstick cooking spray. Put it over medium-high heat. While the skillet's heating, salt and pepper your chops lightly on both sides. When the skillet's hot, add the olive oil, slosh it around to cover the bottom of the skillet, then add the pork chops. Sear them till they're golden brown on both sides.

Add the chicken broth, vermouth, and thyme to the skillet. Cover, turn the heat to medium-low, and let the chops simmer for 10 minutes, until cooked through but not dry.

Transfer the chops to plates. Turn the heat back up to medium-high under the skillet. Add the mustard and lemon juice and stir till the sauce is smooth and cooked down to the thickness of cream. Pour the sauce over the chops and serve.

4 servings, each with 339 calories, 24 g fat, 27 g protein, 1 g carbohydrate, trace fiber

I-Love-Peg-Bracken Pork Chops

For the uninitiated, Peg Bracken wrote the bestselling cookbook of the 1960s, *The I Hate to Cook Book*, and several sequels. Not only were her recipes both uncomplicated and tasty, but her cookbooks were hilarious, worth reading just for the fun of it. I unabashedly admit that Peg is my idol, and I have adapted several of her recipes in my career. This recipe is one. I left out the flour, added onions and the chicken broth, and changed the preparation a little, but the flavors are hers.

> 1 teaspoon seasoned salt
> 1 teaspoon celery salt
> 1 teaspoon powdered garlic
> 2 teaspoons paprika
> 2 pounds pork loin chops, in 4 servings
> 1 tablespoon olive oil, or a little more if you need it
> 2 small apples (I use Granny Smith)
> 2 green bell peppers
> 2 medium onions
> ⅔ cup chicken broth
> 2 tablespoons Worcestershire sauce
> 1½ tablespoons Sucanat *or* 1½ tablespoons Splenda and
> ¼ teaspoon blackstrap molasses
> Guar or xanthan

First stir together the first four ingredients. Lay your chops out on a platter or cutting board and sprinkle this mixture all over both sides of them. Use it all up.

Put the biggest darned skillet you can get your hands on over medium heat. Add the olive oil and sear your chops on both sides till they're golden all over. You may have to do this in two batches.

While your chops are browning, core and slice your apples (don't bother to peel them) and peppers and slice your onions.

Mix together the broth, Worcestershire sauce, and Sucanat or Splenda and molasses.

When your chops are brown, remove them from the pan and put them on a platter or chopping board. Throw the apples, peppers, and onions into the skillet and sauté them for 4–5minutes, stirring frequently. Then spread them evenly in the pan.

Place the chops on top—you may have to stack them. Pour the broth mixture over everything. Now cover the skillet, turn the burner to low, and simmer for 40 minutes.

When time's up, transfer the chops to a platter or to serving plates. Use your guar or xanthan shaker to thicken up the liquid in the skillet to about heavy cream texture. Pile all the apples, peppers, and onions on top of the chops, pour the liquid over everything, and serve.

4 servings, each with 367 calories, 16 g fat, 30 g protein, 24 g carbohydrate, 4 g fiber

Pork Ribs Adobado

My husband and I love spareribs, but I'm not one of those barbecue fanatics willing to run out to the Weber in the snow. These ribs roast in the oven. They take time but are quite simple, and the results are so worth it.

> 2 teaspoons garlic powder
> 1 tablespoon paprika
> 1 teaspoon ground cumin
> 1 teaspoon dried oregano
> 1 teaspoon salt or Vege-Sal
> ½ teaspoon pepper
> 3 pounds pork spareribs
> ½ cup chicken broth or beer
> 3 tablespoons olive oil

Preheat the oven to 325°F.

In a small dish, stir together the seasonings. Transfer 1 tablespoon of the mixture to a cereal bowl and reserve.

Spray a roasting pan with nonstick cooking spray and throw in your slab of ribs. Sprinkle them all over with the seasoning mixture that you didn't reserve in the cereal bowl. Get all sides. Then stick 'em in the oven and set your timer for 25 minutes (or 20 or 30; timing is not extra-critical here).

While the ribs are roasting, stir the chicken broth or beer and the olive oil into the reserved rub.

When the timer goes off, baste your ribs with the broth/olive oil mop, turning them over as you do so. Stick 'em back in the oven and set the timer for another 20 minutes.

Repeat, for a good 1½ to 2 hours; you want your ribs sizzling brown all over and tender when you pierce them with a fork. Cut into individual ribs to serve.

6 servings, each with 474 calories, 40 g fat, 25 g protein, 2 g carbohydrate, trace fiber

Quasi-Cambodian Ribs

I started with a recipe for Cambodian pork kabobs and a package of country-style ribs. I substituted here and there for ingredients I didn't have on hand—hence the *quasi*—and didn't bother to cut up the meat and put it on skewers. The results were fabulous.

2½ pounds pork country-style ribs
¼ cup lime juice
2 tablespoons grated fresh ginger
2 tablespoons ground turmeric
2 tablespoons chili garlic paste, or to taste
2 tablespoons fish sauce
2 tablespoons natural peanut butter
¼ cup coconut milk
¼ cup Splenda or Sucanat
¼ small onion

Lay your ribs in a nonreactive pan or put them in a gallon-size resealable plastic bag.

Put everything else in your blender or food processor with the S-blade in place and run till it's smooth.

Pour the marinade over the ribs, turning to coat. Stick the whole thing in the fridge and let 'em marinate for at least a few hours; overnight is great.

When it's time to cook, pull out your bag of ribs and drain off the marinade into a bowl. Arrange your ribs on your broiler rack (give it a shot of nonstick cooking spray first) and broil 4–6 inches from the heat. Every 12–15 minutes, turn your ribs over, basting them with the reserved marinade. If some are cooking faster than others, use tongs to switch the ribs around to even things out. It'll take about 1 to 1¼ hours total—poke 'em with a fork and see if the juices run clear and they feel tender.

Put any remaining marinade in a saucepan and boil it hard for a minute or two to kill the raw pork germs, then serve as a dipping sauce with the ribs.

5 servings, each with 478 calories, 36 g fat, 28 g protein, 9 g carbohydrate, 1 g fiber

Soy and Sesame Pork Steak

Shoulder steaks are my favorite cut of pork. I've been known to eat them three days running!

> 2 tablespoons soy sauce
> ½ teaspoon dark sesame oil
> 2 teaspoons Splenda or Sucanat
> ½ teaspoon chili garlic paste
> 8 ounces pork shoulder steak, about ¼ inch thick
> 2 teaspoons coconut oil or olive oil

Mix together the soy sauce, sesame oil, Splenda or Sucanat, and chili garlic paste. Lay your pork steak on a plate with a rim and pour this mixture over it, turning to coat. Let it sit for 15 minutes or so.

Give your big skillet a shot of nonstick cooking spray and put it over medium-high heat. Melt the oil. Now throw in your pork steak.

Give it 5–7 minutes on each side—you want it browned on the outside and done through but not dried out.

Pour any leftover marinade from the plate over the cooked steak in the skillet. Flip once or twice, cooking for another 30 to 60 seconds on each side, to let the heat kill any germs; then serve.

2 servings, each with 262 calories, 21 g fat, 16 g protein, 2 g carbohydrate, trace fiber

Pork with Lemon-Scallion Topping

Bright, sunny flavor!

> 1 tablespoon olive oil
> 1 pound pork shoulder steaks or thin pork chops
> ¼ cup lemon juice
> 4 teaspoons soy sauce
> 4 teaspoons Splenda or sugar
> 12 scallions, including the crisp greens, sliced thin
> Salt and pepper to taste

Give your big, heavy skillet a shot of nonstick cooking spray; then put it over medium heat. Add the oil and slosh it around. When the pan is hot, throw in your pork steaks. Let them cook through, turning once; they should be nicely browned on both sides.

While the pork is cooking, stir together your lemon juice, soy sauce, and Splenda.

Transfer the steaks to serving plates. Now add the lemon juice mixture and scallions to the skillet and stir around, scraping up any tasty browned bits from the bottom. Let the mixture cook down till it's slightly syrupy. Pour over the pork, scraping the pan to get all of it, and serve.

3 servings, each with 339 calories, 25 g fat, 21 g protein, 8 g carbohydrate, 2 g fiber

Southwestern Pork with Peach Salsa

Boneless pork loin is so lean it can be bland. Not here!

> 2 tablespoons olive oil
> 1½ pounds boneless pork loin, sliced ½ inch thick
> ¼ cup chicken broth
> 2 teaspoons chili powder
> ½ teaspoon minced garlic
> ¼ teaspoon ground cumin
> 1 tablespoon dry white wine
> 2 tablespoons lime juice
> 1 chipotle chile canned in adobo
> ⅔ cup frozen peach slices
> ⅓ cucumber
> ¼ medium red onion
> ½ jalapeño pepper
> 2 teaspoons rice vinegar
> 1 dash Tabasco sauce
> Salt to taste

In your big, heavy skillet, heat the olive oil over medium-high heat. Add the pork and brown it lightly on both sides.

While that's happening, combine the chicken broth, chili powder, garlic, cumin, wine, and lime juice. Chop the chipotle. When the pork is golden on both sides, pour the chicken broth mixture into the skillet and stir in the chipotle. Turn the heat to medium and let the mixture simmer, uncovered, for 6 or 7 minutes.

Meanwhile, put the peach slices, cucumber, onion, jalapeño, vinegar, and Tabasco into your food processor with the S-blade in place and pulse until everything is chopped medium-fine. Add the salt and pulse once or twice more.

Go turn over your pork! Let it simmer for another 5–6 minutes. Serve with some of the pan liquid and the peach salsa on top.

4 servings, each with 316 calories, 15 g fat, 32 g protein, 13 g carbohydrate, 2 g fiber

Sausage, Wild Rice, and Cranberry Skillet Supper

The wild rice adds a true grain flavor without adding a ton of starch. And as my husband put it, "The dried cranberries really make the whole thing!"

> 1 pound bulk pork sausage (use turkey sausage
>   if you prefer)
> ½ head cauliflower
> 8 ounces sliced mushrooms—portobello, if you can get
>   'em, but good old button mushrooms will do
> 1 cup chopped onion
> ¾ cup shredded carrot
> 2 teaspoons chicken bouillon concentrate
> ½ cup cooked wild rice
> ⅓ cup dried cranberries
> ½ cup chopped fresh parsley
> 2 teaspoons poultry seasoning

Put your biggest skillet over medium heat and start browning and crumbling your sausage.

Trim the leaves and the base of the stem from your cauliflower. Whack the rest into chunks and run 'em through your food processor's shredding disk. Put the resulting "rice" into a microwavable casserole with a lid. Add a tablespoon or two of water, cover, and nuke on high for 6 minutes.

By now some fat has cooked out of your sausage. Throw in the mushrooms, onion, and carrot and keep cooking everything together.

When the microwave beeps, uncover your cauliflower right away! Otherwise, it'll become mush.

OK, the pink color is gone from the sausage, the mushrooms have changed color, and the onion is translucent. Drain off any extra grease. Now dump in the "rice"—don't bother to drain it first.

Add the bouillon concentrate and stir till it dissolves. Now stir in everything else. Let the whole thing cook for another minute or two and serve.

4 servings, each with 544 calories, 46 g fat, 17 g protein, 16 g carbohydrate, 3 g fiber

Note: Wild rice has 25 percent less starch than brown rice and a whole lot more flavor, making it a good addition to our " rice." It comes in teeny boxes in the rice aisle at the grocery store. Be careful to get just wild rice, not "wild and long-grain rice blend" or the like. Cook it according to package directions and freeze it in a snap-top container. Then you'll always have it on hand for quick use.

Slow-Cooker Ham Dinner

Everyone loves ham, but it's not the sort of thing you can make on a weeknight. It just takes too darned long. Your slow-cooker to the rescue! (This takes a big slow-cooker, though.)

> 5 medium turnips
> 2 pounds cabbage
> 5 pounds ham (this will be ½ ham)
> 1 cup chicken broth

Peel your turnips and cut 'em into eighths. Throw 'em into your slow-cooker. Core your cabbage and cut it into chunks and throw it in too.

Now nestle your ham down among all those veggies. It'll take a little doing to fit it down far enough for the lid to go on the slow-cooker; you may have to make a hole in the veggies. Mine fits best curved end down, flat cut surface up. When your ham is in far enough that you can put the lid on the slow-cooker, pour in the chicken broth, slap on the lid, and set the sucker to low. Forget about it for 8 hours.

When dinnertime rolls around, lift out the ham and put it on a platter. Using a slotted spoon, fish out the veggies and pile them around the ham, and serve. Butter is good on the vegetables, but they'll be flavorful without it.

10 servings, each with 461 calories, 30 g fat, 38 g protein, 9 g carbohydrate, 3 g fiber

Slow-Cooker Southwestern Pork Roast

You may find shoulder roast labeled *picnic roast.* Where I live they often go on sale for 99 cents a pound!

> **3 pounds pork shoulder roast**
> **2 tablespoons olive oil**
> **2 large carrots, cut into chunks**
> **2 large onions, cut into eighths**
> **Salt and pepper to taste**
> **1 teaspoon dried oregano**
> **1 teaspoon ground cumin**
> **½ teaspoon ground coriander**
> **2 cloves garlic, minced**
> **¾ cup light beer**

Remove any skin from the roast. Put your big, heavy skillet over medium heat and get it good and hot. Add the oil and throw your pork roast in. You're going to sear it on all sides till it's good and brown.

While your roast is searing, put your carrots and onions in the bottom of your slow-cooker.

When the roast is brown all over, salt and pepper it on all sides. Sprinkle the oregano, cumin, and coriander evenly over all sides of the roast too. Place your roast on top of the veggies in your slow-cooker. Scatter the garlic over the roast—you want most of it on top of the roast, with a little falling down into the veggies below.

Pour the light beer around the roast, not over it; you don't want to wash the seasonings off. Cover the slow-cooker and set to low. Cook for 7–8 hours.

8 servings, each with 359 calories, 27 g fat, 23 g protein, 5 g carbohydrate, 1 g fiber

Slow-Cooker Sesame Ribs

Talk about falling-off-the-bone tender! If you love the spareribs at Chinese restaurants, you must try this.

>   3 pounds pork spareribs
>   1 cup Splenda (use sugar if you must, but it's a lot)
>   ½ cup ketchup
>   2 tablespoons cider vinegar
>   3 cloves garlic, peeled and crushed
>   1 tablespoon grated fresh ginger
>   1 teaspoon chili garlic paste
>   1 tablespoon dark sesame oil
>   2 tablespoons soy sauce
>   1 small onion, sliced

Cut your slab of ribs into three shorter lengths. Lay them on your broiler rack and slide 'em under the broiler, close to the heat. Give them about 10 minutes per side—you want them browned and crisp on both sides.

While your ribs are browning, mix together everything else but the onion.

Slice the onion and put it in the bottom of your slow-cooker. Pour a little of the sauce over them. Now lay a section of ribs on the onion and pour some more sauce on it. Spread it over the surface. Lay another section of ribs on top of the first and spread more sauce on that. Top with the final section of ribs and the rest of the sauce.

Cover, set on low, and let cook for 6–8 hours. Serve with plenty of napkins!

5 servings, each with 568 calories, 43 g fat, 30 g protein, 15 g carbohydrate, 1 g fiber

Indian Lamb Skillet Supper

This exotic and wonderful dish is a great illustration of how you can use cauliflower "rice" in place of starchy grain in all sorts of skillet suppers.

> 12 ounces ground lamb
> ½ large head cauliflower
> ½ medium onion
> 2 cloves garlic, minced
> 2 tablespoons minced fresh mint
> 1 tablespoon minced fresh cilantro
> 1 teaspoon grated fresh ginger
> ¾ teaspoon beef bouillon concentrate
> ¾ teaspoon chicken bouillon concentrate
> ½ teaspoon ground turmeric
> ½ teaspoon ground cumin
> 1 tablespoon lime juice
> 1 teaspoon Splenda or sugar

Put your big, heavy skillet over medium heat and start the lamb browning.

Meanwhile, trim the leaves and the very bottom of the stem from your cauliflower and whack it into hunks. Run through the shredding blade of your food processor. Go stir the lamb!

Dump your shredded cauliflower into a microwavable casserole with a lid. Add a couple of tablespoons of water, cover, and microwave on high for 6 minutes.

By now some fat has cooked out of your lamb. Add the onion and garlic and continue cooking and crumbling until all the pink is gone from the lamb and the onion is translucent.

When the microwave beeps, pull your cauliflower out, uncover immediately to stop the cooking, and drain. Add to the lamb and onion mixture.

Stir in the mint, cilantro, ginger, bouillon concentrates, turmeric, and cumin. Stir till everything is well distributed and the bouillon concentrate is dissolved.

In a small dish, stir the lime juice and Splenda or sugar together, add, and stir in. Make sure everything is seasoned evenly and serve.

I've been known to add a teeny bit of hot sauce to my serving, but that's hardly essential.

3 servings, each with 361 calories, 27 g fat, 21 g protein, 9 g carbohydrate, 3 g fiber

Orange-Rosemary-Glazed Lamb Chops

I love lamb chops, but they're pricey. So I also make this recipe with lamb steaks instead. When whole legs of lamb are on sale, I have the nice meat guys cut a chunk off either end for small roasts and slice the rest ¾ inch thick for steaks. These lamb steaks are lean, meaty, and wonderful—and cheaper than lamb chops!

> 1½ pounds lamb chops or lamb leg steaks, in 4 portions
> 2 tablespoons spicy brown mustard
> 1 tablespoon olive oil
> 2 tablespoons low-sugar orange preserves
> ¼ cup dry white wine
> ½ teaspoon ground rosemary
> 1 teaspoon lemon juice
> ½ teaspoon Splenda or sugar

Give your big, heavy skillet a shot of nonstick cooking spray and put it over medium heat.

While the pan is heating, spread ½ teaspoon of mustard over each side of each of your chops, using 4 teaspoons mustard total.

OK, the pan is hot. Add the olive oil and throw in your chops.

While the chops are browning, mix together the rest of the mustard, the orange preserves, wine, rosemary, lemon juice, and Splenda.

Time to flip your lamb chops! Cook 'em good and brown on the outside, but leave 'em pink in the middle. Transfer to serving plates.

Now pour the preserves mixture into the skillet and mix it around, scraping up any brown crusty bits on the skillet. Let it cook down till it's syrupy, pour it over the chops, and serve.

4 servings, each with 475 calories, 40 g fat, 23 g protein, 4 g carbohydrate, trace fiber

Slow-Cooker Lamb Shanks

Tough, cheap, flavorful lamb shanks are perfect for slow cooking. They come out fork-tender and utterly delicious. With Fauxtatoes (Chapter 6) they're scrumptious.

> 1 tablespoon olive oil
> 2 pounds lamb shanks—2 good-sized shanks,
>   but be sure they'll fit into your slow-cooker!
> 2 medium onions, sliced
> 8 ounces sliced mushrooms
> ¼ cup dry white wine
> ¼ cup tomato sauce
> ½ teaspoon paprika
> ½ teaspoon ground ginger
> ½ teaspoon beef bouillon concentrate
> ½ teaspoon pepper
> ½ cup chicken broth
> Guar or xanthan

Coat your big, heavy skillet with nonstick cooking spray and put it over medium-high heat. Add the olive oil and throw in your lamb shanks. You're searing them. You want to get them good and brown all over their surface.

While the lamb shanks are searing, haul out your slow-cooker and throw in the onions and mushrooms. Stir together everything else but the guar or xanthan (be sure the bouillon is dissolved).

When the shanks are nicely browned, put them in the slow-cooker on top of the veggies. Pour the sauce over everything, cover the pot, set it for low, and let it cook for 8–10 hours.

When it's time to serve, pull out the lamb shanks and throw them on a platter. Use your guar or xanthan shaker to thicken up the sauce just a tad—maybe the texture of cream.

Carve each shank into two portions of meat and serve with Fauxtatoes, piling the onions and mushrooms over everything and pouring the sauce over it all. YUM!

4 servings, each with 452 calories, 28 g fat, 36 g protein, 9 g carbohydrate, 2 g fiber (analysis does not include Fauxtatoes)

11

Fish and Seafood

ish has long been considered the healthiest of animal foods. It's true that fish is a great source of protein and often of good fats as well. It has the added advantage of cooking quickly.

But we've learned that some of what made fish look so healthy compared to red meat was that, until recently, most of it was wild-caught, not farmed. Turns out that feeding grains and beans to fish causes the same kinds of shifts in fatty acid profiles as we see in grain-fed beef. Doesn't make fish bad for you—but it does mean that wild-caught fish are worth paying extra for if your budget will stretch.

Seared Fish with Ginger-Lime Cucumber Topping

This is nothing short of amazing, and it's so quick and easy. The cucumber shreds hold the sauce on the fish and add a cool note of their own. You have to try this!

> Ginger-Lime Dipping Sauce (recipe follows)
> ½ cucumber
> 1 tablespoon coconut oil or peanut oil
> Salt and pepper to taste
> 18 ounces fish fillets—sea bass, red snapper,
>   orange roughy, sole, flounder, or tilapia

First make your dipping sauce, which is extremely easy. Now use the tip of a spoon to scrape the seeds out of your cucumber half. Run the cucumber flesh through the shredding disk of your food processor or shred it on a box grater. Either way, try to get the longest strands you can. (In your food processor, this means laying chunks of cuke down in the feed tube so they get shredded the long way, instead of across.) Gather up your shredded cuke and plunk it into your bowl of dipping sauce.

OK, it's time to cook your fish. Give your big, heavy skillet a shot of nonstick cooking spray and put it over medium-high heat. Let it get hot, then add your oil and slosh it around to coat the skillet. Salt and pepper your fillets on both sides and throw them into the fat. Give them about 5 minutes per side—you want them done through but not dry and nicely browned on both sides. Transfer to serving plates.

Using a fork (or, heck, clean fingers!) fish the cucumber strands out of the dipping sauce and divide them equally among the fillets, piling them on top. Use 'em all! Drizzle a little more of the sauce from the dish over each fillet and serve immediately.

3 servings, each with 222 calories, 7 g fat, 31 g protein, 7 g carbohydrate, 1 g fiber

Ginger-Lime Dipping Sauce

This would be good with a sautéed chicken breast too.

 2 tablespoons grated fresh ginger
 2 garlic cloves, peeled and crushed
 2 tablespoons Splenda or sugar
 ½ lime, juiced
 2 tablespoons water
 2 tablespoons fish sauce (nuoc mam or nam pla)
 ½ teaspoon chili garlic paste, or to taste

Just mix everything together!

4 servings, each with 28 calories, 1 g fat, trace protein, 4 g carbohydrate, trace fiber

Baked Perch in Roasted Red Pepper–Sun-Dried Tomato Sauce

This quick and easy recipe drew raves from dinner party company.

1½ pounds ocean perch fillets
2 tablespoons lemon juice
Salt and pepper to taste
1 cup roasted red peppers jarred in water, drained
1 cup drained oil-packed sun-dried tomatoes
½ cup dry white wine
1 small onion, quartered
2 cloves garlic, chopped
1 teaspoon Creole seasoning (Tony Chachere's is good)

Preheat the oven to 350°F.

Spray a nonreactive shallow baking dish (glass, enamel, stainless steel) with nonstick cooking spray. Lay the perch fillets skin side down in the prepared baking dish. Sprinkle with the lemon juice and salt and pepper them. Set aside.

Put all the other ingredients in your food processor with the S-blade in place and pulse till the peppers, sun-dried tomatoes, and onion are chopped medium-fine. Spoon the resulting sauce evenly over the fish fillets.

Bake uncovered for 20–25 minutes, transfer to plates, and serve.

6 servings, each with 175 calories, 5 g fat, 23 g protein, 8 g carbohydrate, 2 g fiber

Easy and Elegant Salmon Packets

Exactly what the name says—and no pan to wash!

> **1 pound salmon fillet in 4 servings**
> **Salt and pepper to taste**
> **8 thin lemon slices**
> **4 sprigs fresh dill**
> **2 tablespoons dry vermouth**

Preheat the oven to 375°F.

Tear off four roughly 12-inch squares of foil. Lay a salmon fillet in the middle of each. Salt and pepper them.

Now cover each fillet with two thin lemon slices and top with a sprig of dill. Sprinkle ½ tablespoon vermouth over each.

Fold up the sides of the foil and roll down. Then roll up the ends. Place the packets on a pan, in case of leaks, and bake for 20–25 minutes. Serve in foil, letting diners open their own packets.

4 servings, each with 147 calories, 4 g fat, 23 g protein, 3 g carbohydrate, trace fiber

Bass with Sour Cream–Roasted Red Pepper Sauce

With a salad of spinach or mixed baby greens in a simple vinaigrette, you've got a dinner any restaurant would be proud of—in less than a half hour, tops!

> **Salt and pepper to taste**
> **1½ pounds sea bass fillets in 4 servings**
> **2 tablespoons lemon juice**
> **½ teaspoon dried thyme**
> **½ cup light sour cream**
> **1 teaspoon Dijon or spicy brown mustard**
> **1 teaspoon ketchup**
> **2 tablespoons diced roasted red pepper jarred in water**
> **2 scallions, including the crisp greens, minced**

Preheat the oven to 400°F. Spray a casserole dish that has a lid with nonstick cooking spray. (If you don't have a covered casserole that fits your fillets, you can use a glass baking pan and cover it tightly with foil.)

Lightly salt and pepper your bass fillets and lay them in the casserole. Sprinkle the lemon juice and thyme over them. Cover the casserole and place in the oven. Bake for 8–10 minutes.

While your fish is baking, stir together the sour cream, mustard, ketchup, diced roasted red pepper, and one of the minced scallions.

Uncover the fish. Spread the sour cream mixture evenly over the fillets and replace the fish in the oven. Bake for 2–3 more minutes.

Serve the bass with the second minced scallion scattered over it for garnish.

4 servings, each with 214 calories, 7 g fat, 33 g protein, 4 g carbohydrate, 1 g fiber

Caramelized Shrimp

This is Vietnamese in inspiration. It's supposed to be three servings, but my husband has been known to devour a whole pound of these on his own.

2 tablespoons peanut oil or coconut oil
1 pound large E-Z peel shrimp
1½ tablespoons Sucanat *or* 1½ tablespoons Splenda plus ⅛ teaspoon blackstrap molasses (or the darkest available)
1 clove garlic, peeled and crushed
1 shallot, minced
¼ cup water
1 tablespoon fish sauce (nuoc mam or nam pla)
¼ teaspoon salt
¼ cup minced fresh cilantro

Have everything prepped and ready to go before you start cooking.

Put your biggest skillet over medium heat and add your oil. When it's hot, throw in the shrimp. Sprinkle the Sucanat or Splenda and molasses over them and stir-fry for 1 minute.

Add the garlic and shallot and stir-fry for another minute. Now add the water, fish sauce, and salt. Turn the heat down to medium-low and let the shrimp cook for another minute or two, till the pan is just about dry and the shrimp are cooked through.

Plate your shrimp, top each with a tablespoon of minced cilantro, and serve with big piles of napkins!

3 servings, each with 240 calories, 11 g fat, 25 g protein, 9 g carbohydrate, trace fiber

Grilled Herb and Garlic Shrimp

This makes a great main course, but would also work well as a crowd-pleasing appetizer.

> ¼ cup lemon juice
> ½ cup olive oil
> 1½ tablespoons Italian seasoning
> 16 cloves garlic, peeled and crushed
> 1½ tablespoons paprika
> ¼ teaspoon hot red pepper flakes
> ½ teaspoon black pepper
> ¼ teaspoon salt
> 2½ tablespoons Sucanat
> 2 pounds large peeled shrimp (2 or 3 ounces more if they're in the shell)

Mix together everything but your shrimp. This is your marinade.

If your shrimp aren't peeled, peel 'em. Throw your peeled shrimp into a nonreactive bowl or a resealable plastic bag. Dump the marinade on top and stir them up till they're coated with the stuff. Now stash them in the fridge for a couple hours or all day if you like.

When suppertime rolls around, you have a decision to make: You can cook these over your backyard grill. You can throw your marinated shrimp in your electric tabletop grill for 2½–3 minutes—that's what I do. Or you could broil 'em close to the heat for a minute or so per side. Up to you. Whatever you do, don't overcook!

4 servings, each with 482 calories, 29 g fat, 39 g protein, 16 g carbohydrate, 1 g fiber

Asian Steamed Scallops

I made this in little heatproof ramekins, but if you have nice decorative scallop shells, use them instead—though they'll be harder to fit into your steamer! (If you don't own a steamer, bamboo ones are available cheaply at Asian markets and import stores.) As it is, you may need to do this in two batches.

This would also make a good appetizer for eight—one scallop per serving instead of two.

>1 pound sea scallops—about 8 very large scallops
>Salt and pepper to taste
>8 thin slices fresh ginger, plus 2 tablespoons grated
>6 scallions
>4 cloves garlic
>½ teaspoon chili paste
>¼ cup soy sauce
>4 teaspoons dark sesame oil
>2 teaspoons water
>1½ teaspoons Splenda

Start water heating in a pot that will fit your steamer.

Put two scallops each into four small heatproof dishes. Salt and pepper them lightly.

Use a sharp knife to cut your ginger slices into skinny little strips, the thinner the better. Trim the roots off the scallions and any wilted parts of the green tops. Now separate the crisp green part from the white part. Cut the green part lengthwise into long, skinny strips. Whack the white parts into two or three pieces each.

Whack the garlic cloves with the flat side of your knife to loosen the skin. Pick the skin off and then mince one clove fine.

Scatter the skinny strips of ginger and scallion greens, plus the minced garlic, over the scallops, dividing them equally.

By now your water should be boiling. Put the dishes in your steamer and put the steamer over the boiling water. Cover and steam for 10–12 minutes, until the scallops are opaque and have firmed up.

While that's happening, put the white parts of the scallions and the remaining cloves of garlic into your food processor with the S-blade in place. Add everything else, including the grated ginger, and whirl till the cloves and scallion are minced fine. This is your sauce.

When the scallops are done, put each dish on a small plate, with a little puddle of the sauce for dipping, and serve.

4 servings, each with 223 calories, 7 g fat, 27 g protein, 11 g carbohydrate, 1 g fiber

Catfish with Browned Butter and Mustard Sauce

Catfish is inexpensive and very flavorful, so I keep trying new ways of cooking it! This is fast and easy, and the sour cream–mustard sauce adds a richness not usually found in sautéed fish.

2½ tablespoons Worcestershire sauce, or as needed
18 ounces catfish fillets
1½ tablespoons butter
1½ tablespoons olive oil
¼ cup sour cream
1½ teaspoons brown mustard

Put 2 tablespoons of the Worcestershire on a plate with a rim and drop your catfish into it; turn it over to coat both sides. Let it sit there for a minute while you . . .

Give your big, heavy skillet a dose of nonstick cooking spray and put it over medium heat. Add the butter and olive oil and slosh 'em together as the butter melts. Let them cook together till you see the little bit of foam from the butter turning brown.

Now pull your catfish out of the Worcestershire, letting the excess drip off, and throw it into the hot fat. Cook, pressing down with your spatula from time to time to minimize curling, for 5–7 minutes per side, or till done through.

While the fish is cooking, during one of those moments when you're not pressing down with your spatula, measure and mix together the sour cream, mustard, and remaining Worcestershire sauce.

When the fish is flaky clear through, put it on serving plates and top each fillet with a dollop of mustard sauce. Serve!

3 servings, each with 326 calories, 22 g fat, 29 g protein, 3 g carbohydrate, trace fiber

Deviled Catfish

Catfish is usually dredged in cornmeal and deep-fried in questionable fat—tasty, but not exactly great for you. Mixing cornmeal and almond meal keeps the flavor and the crunch while lowering the glycemic load.

> ¼ cup whole-grain cornmeal
> ½ cup almond meal
> 1 teaspoon Old Bay seasoning (you'll find this in the
>   spice aisle)
> ¼ cup brown mustard
> 1½ tablespoons Tabasco sauce
> 1 tablespoon coconut oil
> 1 tablespoon olive oil
> 1 pound catfish nuggets or fillets

On a plate, mix together the cornmeal, almond meal, and Old Bay seasoning. In a dish, mix together the mustard and hot sauce.

Give your big, heavy skillet a squirt of nonstick cooking spray and put it over medium-high heat. Add the coconut oil and olive oil and start them heating; slosh them together as the coconut oil melts.

Dip your catfish nuggets in the mustard/hot sauce mixture, using a fork to turn till coated well. Then drop into the corn/almond meal mixture, again turning to coat. As they're coated, drop each nugget in the hot fat and fry till crispy all over, turning to brown. Serve hot!

4 servings, each with 280 calories, 15 g fat, 27 g protein, 12 g carbohydrate, 1 g fiber

Creamed Tuna with Noodles

Remember that tuna-noodle casserole your mom used to make with the canned cream of mushroom soup and the peas? The one that was so humble, homey, comfy—and yummy? This is a dead ringer—but with the starchy stuff cut out.

> 1 tablespoon butter
> ½ medium onion, chopped
> 2 cups chopped mushrooms
> 1 cup frozen peas
> 12 ounces canned tuna in water, drained
> 1½ cups half-and-half
> 1½ teaspoons Worcestershire sauce
> 1 teaspoon beef bouillon concentrate
> 16 ounces tofu shirataki noodles (fettuccine width)
> Salt and pepper to taste

In a big saucepan over medium-low heat, melt your butter and start sautéing the onion and mushrooms.

While that's happening, put your peas, still frozen, in a microwavable bowl. Add a tablespoon or so of water, cover with a plate or saucer, and nuke for 4 minutes on high.

When the mushrooms have softened and changed color, and the onion is translucent, drain the peas and dump them into the pan. Drain your tuna and add it too. Pour in your half-and-half and stir in the Worcestershire and bouillon concentrate. Let the whole thing come to a simmer, stirring now and then. When your mixture is at a simmer, adjust the heat to keep it there (instead of boiling hard) and let it simmer for 8–10 minutes.

Meanwhile, snip open your shirataki packets and drain them. When the 8–10 minutes are up, dump in the noodles and stir them in. Salt and pepper to taste and serve.

4 servings, each with 303 calories, 14 g fat, 31 g protein, 12 g carbohydrate, 2 g fiber

Note: *Buy chunk light tuna rather than the more expensive white—i.e., albacore—tuna. It has far less mercury.*

Hot Tuna Wraps

I tried heating these in my electric tabletop grill, but the filling squeezed out all over the place! So heat them in the oven.

> 1 6-ounce can tuna in water, drained
> 2 ounces Swiss cheese, diced
> 2 ounces sharp cheddar cheese, diced
> 3 hard-boiled eggs, peeled and chopped
> ¼ medium green bell pepper, diced small
> ¼ medium onion, diced small
> 2 tablespoons chopped pimiento-stuffed green olives
> 2 tablespoons sweet pickle relish
> ¼ cup light mayonnaise
> 5 large low-carb tortillas

Preheat the oven to 350°F. Drain the tuna and dump it into a mixing bowl. Flake it up thoroughly with a fork. Add everything else but the tortillas and mix well.

Lay a large tortilla on a plate and put 3 rounded tablespoons of the tuna mixture on it. Fold up the bottom, then fold in the sides and roll. Place the filled tortillas seam side down on a baking sheet and bake for 20 minutes. Serve hot.

5 servings, each with 298 calories, 16 g fat, 19 g protein, 24 g carbohydrate, 14 g fiber

12

Desserts

have mixed feelings about this chapter. I have a history of serious sugar addiction. I've been known to eat a pound of milk chocolate, a pound of hard candies, and four or five ice-cream sandwiches all in one day. I used to steal money from my parents' wallets to buy those outrageous quantities of sugary stuff. And there is no question that at those levels sugary foods have a high-glycemic load.

So be aware: a few squares of chocolate or a half-dozen jelly beans after a meal will not jack up your glycemic load. But if you take this to mean that so long as you don't eat starches, you can chow down on all the starch-free sweets you want, you're fooling yourself. Remember our equation: *glycemic load = glycemic index × grams of carbohydrate.*

Only you know where your demons lie. Be honest with yourself about what you can handle. If you can eat a little sugar without having it turn into a lot of sugar, go ahead, but remember to avoid sweets that mix sugar with starch, like cakes, cookies, pies, and puddings. Eat sweets at the end of a meal. It's a good rule not to eat sugar on an empty stomach or to quell hunger.

So what can you have?

A few squares of chocolate, the darker the better
A couple of truffles!
Chocolate-dipped strawberries. Because the berries
    themselves are quite low in sugar, you can afford to eat
    four or five!
A few chocolate-covered nuts of any kind, including peanut
    M&Ms
A handful of chocolate-covered coffee beans
One or two pieces of hard candy
A small piece of peanut brittle
A small handful of jelly beans
One "fun-size" Snickers bar
Two or three mini peanut butter cups
Super-premium ice cream, the richer the better. Choose
    a variety without chunks of starchy, sugary stuff like
    cookie dough or brownie. Plain chocolate, chocolate-
    almond, vanilla, coffee, and the like are good. We
    both feel that ice cream has strong potential to trigger
    bingeing. If you can't limit yourself to a single scoop at a
    time, skip it. Or have an ice-cream bar instead.

For the following recipes, I've walked the middle path where
sugar is concerned. I've used some Sucanat and some Splenda,
while concentrating on keeping total carb load low.

Dr. Rob Says: How Sugar Can Be Your Friend

*You can't taste starch. Enzymes in your saliva break a
tiny fraction of the starch you eat down to sugar, which
you can taste, but otherwise it's flavorless. However, as
soon as it hits your stomach, it turns to sugar. Scientists
infused sugar through tubes inserted directly into people's*

stomachs and compared their eating behaviors to those of people fed sugar orally. The sugar that people could taste suppressed appetite more than sugar they couldn't taste. People tend to consume more sugar when it is delivered to their bloodstream in the form of starch than they do when it is in the form of table sugar or candy. A good trick for ridding yourself of the urge to eat starch is to finish your meal and have a couple pieces of candy. You might find that you're more satisfied and end up consuming less sugar.

A pile of sugar would raise your blood sugar as much as a similar-size pile of bread, potatoes, or rice. The difference is the serving size. You would never eat as much sugar in one sitting as you would the starch. It's too sweet. The same is true for other candy as long as you can taste all the sugar in it. A few bits of chocolate after dinner can make life enjoyable if you have a sweet tooth and would contribute little to glycemic load.

Coconut Chocolate Chip Cookies

Coconut, long shunned because of its saturated fat, turns out to be remarkably healthful, so I wanted to use it in a cookie—and these are scrumptious.

½ pound (2 sticks) butter at room temperature
1 cup Splenda
½ cup Sucanat
2 eggs
2 cups unsweetened shredded coconut meat
1 cup vanilla whey protein powder
1 teaspoon baking soda
½ teaspoon salt
1½ cups chocolate chips

Preheat the oven to 375°F.

Using your electric mixer, beat the butter till it's creamy and fluffy. Now beat in the Splenda and Sucanat.

Next beat in the eggs, one at a time, beating each one in thoroughly.

In another bowl, mix together the coconut, vanilla whey protein powder, baking soda, and salt till everything is distributed evenly. Now beat this mixture into the butter mixture in three or four additions, beating well after each one.

Finally, stir in the chocolate chips.

Spray your cookie sheets with nonstick cooking spray or line them with baking parchment. Now drop the cookie dough on the cookie sheets—I use a cookie scoop, which is like an ice-cream scoop, only smaller; it holds 2 tablespoons of dough, which makes nice big cookies. If you drop it by smaller spoonfuls, you'll get more, smaller cookies, of course.

Bake for 10–12 minutes, then cool on wire racks.

32 cookies, each with 167 calories, 11 g fat, 6 g protein, 12 g carbohydrate, 1 g fiber. With sugar-free chips: 147 calories, 10 g fat, 6 g protein, 8 g carbohydrates, 3 g fiber. (The extra fiber comes from one of the sugar-free sweeteners.)

Note: *The analysis assumes regular chocolate chips, but I used sugar-free chocolate chips from Carb Smart, an online retailer (carbsmart.com), and they were great.*

Cookie Mix

With this mix in the refrigerator, you're never more than 20 minutes from fresh-baked cookies. Feel free to substitute Splenda for up to two-thirds of the Sucanat in this recipe. If you do, subtract 2 grams of carb from each cookie you make from the mix.

> 1½ pounds (6 sticks) butter
> 3 cups Sucanat
> 1½ cups oat bran
> 1½ cups wheat germ
> 3 cups almond meal
> 3 cups vanilla whey protein powder
> 3 cups powdered milk (the instant skim milk at your grocery store will do fine)
> ¾ cup sesame seeds
> 1 tablespoon salt
> 3 tablespoons baking powder

Put everything in your food processor with the S-blade in place and pulse until the butter is cut in and dispersed evenly. Store in a snap-top container in the fridge or freezer.

Makes a gallon of mix, which will make about 192 cookies, each with 81 calories, 5 g fat, 4 g protein, 6 g carbohydrate, 1 g fiber—until you add other ingredients!

Note: *Buy sesame seeds in bulk at a health food store; they'll be far cheaper than if you buy them in a little bottle off the spice rack. If your health food store offers them, choose unhulled sesame seeds instead of the familiar hulled variety—they're higher in minerals and fiber.*

Here are some ways to use your cookie mix. The directions for all of them are the same:

Preheat the oven to 350°F. Spray a cookie sheet with nonstick cooking spray.

Use your electric mixer to combine everything well. Drop by rounded tablespoonfuls onto the prepared cookie sheet. Bake for 12–15 minutes, then cool on a wire rack.

Almond Cookies from Mix

> 2 cups Cookie Mix
> 1 egg
> ¾ cup almond butter
> 1 teaspoon vanilla extract
> ½ teaspoon almond extract

2 dozen cookies, each with 134 calories, 10 g fat, 5 g protein, 8 g carbohydrate, 1 g fiber

Peanut Butter Cookies from Mix

> 2 cups Cookie Mix
> 1 egg
> ¾ cup natural peanut butter
> 1 teaspoon vanilla extract

2 dozen cookies, each with 131 calories, 9 g fat, 6 g protein, 8 g carbohydrate, 1 g fiber

Sesame Cookies from Mix

> 2 cups Cookie Mix
> 1 egg
> ¾ cup tahini (sesame butter)
> 1 teaspoon vanilla extract

2 dozen cookies, each with 129 calories, 9 g fat, 6 g protein, 8 g carbohydrate, 1 g fiber

Spice Cookies from Mix

>   2 cups Cookie Mix
>   1 egg
>   1 teaspoon ground cinnamon
>   Pinch ground cloves
>   Pinch ground nutmeg
>   1 teaspoon vanilla extract

16 cookies, each with 127 calories, 8 g fat, 6 g protein, 9 g carbohydrate, 1 g fiber

Chocolate Chip Cookies from Mix

>   2 cups Cookie Mix
>   1 egg
>   1 teaspoon vanilla extract
>   ¾ cup chocolate chips

2 dozen cookies, each with 118 calories, 7 g fat, 5 g protein, 10 g carbohydrate, 1 g fiber

"Graham" Crust

Here's what you use instead of a graham cracker crumb crust.

> 2 cups All-Bran, All-Bran Extra Fiber, or
>   Fiber One cereal
> ½ cup raw wheat germ
> ¼ cup Splenda
> 4 tablespoons butter, melted
> 3 tablespoons water

Preheat the oven to 350°F. Spray a pie plate with nonstick cooking spray. (You can use a 9- or a 10-inch pie plate; with the bigger one you'll just get a thinner crust or perhaps not build it up as high on the sides.)

Dump the All-Bran into your food processor (with the S-blade in place) and run till it's ground fine. This took a tad longer than I expected; that All-Bran is sturdy stuff! Don't stop too soon; I did the first time, and while my crust tasted good, the texture left something to be desired.

Add the wheat germ and Splenda and pulse to mix them in.

Add the butter and pulse to mix it in. When the butter is distributed evenly, add the water a tablespoon at a time, pulsing to mix each addition in thoroughly before you add the next.

Turn the mixture into your prepared pie plate and press firmly on the bottom and up the sides.

Bake for 13–15 minutes. Cool before filling.

12 servings, each with 80 calories, 5 g fat, 2 g protein, 11 g carbohydrate, 4 g fiber

Pumpkin Mousse Pie

Fluffy and creamy and festive! And between the pumpkin and the cream, a great source of vitamin A.

> 1 15-ounce can pumpkin
> 1 package instant vanilla pudding and pie filling
>   (I used sugar-free, and it works fine)
> 2 teaspoons ground cinnamon
> ⅛ teaspoon ground cloves
> ⅛ teaspoon ground nutmeg
> 2 cups heavy cream, well chilled
> "Graham" Crust (preceding recipe), baked and
>   ready to go

Scoop the canned pumpkin into a big mixing bowl. Open the pudding mix and set aside 2 tablespoons of the powder. Add the rest to the pumpkin along with the spices. Mix the whole thing up well.

Pour your cream into a deep bowl and add the reserved pudding mix. Use your electric mixer to beat the cream till it's stiff—stands in soft peaks. Add about a third of the whipped cream to the pumpkin and use a rubber scraper to fold it in gently. Fold in another third of the cream, then the final third. Pile the whole thing into your prepared crust and chill for several hours before serving.

12 servings, each with 242 calories, 20 g fat, 4 g protein, 17 g carbohydrate, 5 g fiber (that's with sugar-sweetened pudding mix)

Note: Try making this with a tablespoon of pumpkin pie spice instead of the cinnamon, cloves, and nutmeg.

Lemon-Vanilla Cheesecake

Light, creamy, and lemony. You could top this with fruit if you liked, but it's awfully good as is. Makes a terrific breakfast too.

> 24 ounces creamed cottage cheese
> ½ cup plain yogurt
> 2 eggs
> ¼ cup vanilla whey protein powder
> 1 lemon
> ⅔ cup Splenda
> ¼ teaspoon salt
> 1 "Graham" Crust (see above), made in a 10-inch
> pie plate, baked and ready to go

Preheat the oven to 325°F.

You can make this in your blender or food processor with the S-blade, though I think a food processor works a little better. Either way, process or blend your cottage cheese till it's absolutely smooth.

Add everything else except the crust and process till everything is very well blended.

Pour into your crust. Place in the oven and place another pan with an inch of water in it on the rack below the cake. Bake for 55–60 minutes, then remove from the oven and let cool.

Chill for several hours. Serve by itself or with fruit.

12 servings, each with 180 calories, 9 g fat, 14 g protein, 15 g carbohydrate, 4 g fiber

Applesauce Spice Cake

Wonderful with a cup of tea or coffee. This makes a nice breakfast.

> 1½ cups hulled pumpkin seeds (pepitas)
> 1½ cups vanilla whey protein powder
> 2 teaspoons baking powder
> 1 teaspoon baking soda
> ½ teaspoon salt
> 2 teaspoons ground ginger
> 1½ teaspoons ground cinnamon
> ½ teaspoon ground cloves
> 1½ cups Splenda, Sucanat, or a combination
> 2 cups unsweetened applesauce
> 3 eggs
> ⅓ cup coconut oil, melted
> 1 tablespoon blackstrap molasses

Preheat the oven to 350°F. Spray a nonstick Bundt pan with nonstick cooking spray.

Dump your pumpkin seeds into your food processor with the S-blade in place and grind them to a fine meal. Take a tablespoon or two and sprinkle them over the Bundt pan to "flour" it. Measure the rest; you want 1½ cups pumpkin seed meal. Put it in a mixing bowl.

Add the vanilla whey protein powder, baking powder, baking soda, salt, ginger, cinnamon, cloves, and Splenda. Using a whisk, stir the dry ingredients together till they're distributed evenly.

In another bowl, combine the applesauce, eggs, coconut oil, and blackstrap molasses and whisk them together.

Now dump the wet ingredients into the dry, using a rubber scraper to make sure you get all of the applesauce mixture. Whisk the wet ingredients into the dry, mixing just until you're sure there are no pockets of dry stuff left. Pour your batter into the prepared Bundt pan, again making sure you scrape it all out of the bowl.

Bake for 50–60 minutes, or until a toothpick inserted in the middle between the walls of the cake pan comes out clean. Turn out onto a wire rack to cool.

Serve with a sprinkle of extra Splenda or with whipped cream—or just plain, munched out of your hand, which is how I usually eat it!

18 servings, each with 167 calories, 7 g fat, 16 g protein, 11 g carbohydrate, 2 g fiber

Chocolate Truffle Pie

This is devastating: rich, dense, fudgy, and oh-so-chocolaty. You can use sugar-free dark chocolate if you prefer.

1½ cups pecan halves
¼ cup oat bran
¼ cup vanilla whey protein powder for the crust,
     plus ⅓ cup for the pie
4 tablespoons butter, melted
1 pound semisweet chocolate
1 cup heavy cream
6 eggs
¾ cup Splenda

Preheat the oven to 350°F. Spray a 10-inch pie plate with non-stick cooking spray.

Put your pecans in a roasting pan and slide them into the oven for 10 minutes to toast. Remove them and turn the oven down to 325°F.

Put half the pecans in your food processor (with the S-blade in place) and pulse till they're chopped to a medium consistency. Add the rest of the pecans, the oat bran, and the ¼ cup vanilla whey protein and pulse again till the second batch of pecans is chopped medium fine. Add the butter and pulse just long enough to mix. Turn the mixture into the pie plate and press across the bottom and just a little up the sides.

Put the chocolate and cream in a saucepan and place over the lowest possible heat. (If you have a double boiler or a heat diffuser, use it.)

Meanwhile, put your eggs, ⅓ cup vanilla whey, and Splenda in a mixing bowl and start beating them with an electric mixer. You want to beat them for 10 minutes.

OK, your chocolate is melted and your eggs are done beating. Add about a quarter of the egg mixture to the chocolate and fold it in with a rubber scraper. Now add half the chocolate mixture to the egg, and fold it in; then add the rest of the chocolate and fold it in as well.

Pour the filling into your crust and bake for 45 minutes. Remove from the oven and let it cool, then refrigerate for a few hours before serving. Pull it out of the fridge when you start dinner to take the chill off while you eat. Serve in skinny slices, because how ridiculously rich is this?

16 servings, each with 344 calories, 26 g fat, 11 g protein, 23 g carbohydrate, 1 g fiber

Magic Cake

This is an adaptation of a recipe that was popular back in the 1960s. You could replace the Sucanat with more Splenda if you wanted, but the Sucanat does make for a slightly moister cake. About that powdered egg white: it helps with the texture of flourless baked goods. Find it in the baking aisle of your grocery store.

¾ cup almond meal
¾ cup vanilla whey protein powder
3 tablespoons cocoa powder
½ cup Sucanat
½ cup Splenda
½ teaspoon salt
1 teaspoon baking soda
2 tablespoons powdered egg white
2 teaspoons guar
¼ cup peanut oil
1 tablespoon distilled vinegar
1 cup water

Preheat the oven to 350°F and spray an 8-inch square pan with nonstick cooking spray.

Put the almond meal, protein powder, cocoa powder, Sucanat, Splenda, salt, baking soda, powdered egg white, and guar in your sifter and sift them directly into your prepared pan. Any bits of almond that were too big to go through the strainer can just be dumped on top.

Now make two holes in the sifted mixture. Pour the oil into one and the vinegar into the other.

Pour the water over the whole thing and stir with a spoon until there are no dry bits left. Immediately put in the oven and bake for 30 minutes.

9 servings, each with 239 calories, 12 g fat, 16 g protein, 18 g carbohydrate, 2 g fiber

Old-Fashioned Apple Bars

These taste like something your great-grandma would have made.

½ cup rolled oats
¼ cup wheat germ
¼ cup flaxseed meal
½ cup almond meal
½ cup vanilla whey protein powder
½ teaspoon salt
½ teaspoon ground cinnamon
8 tablespoons (1 stick) butter
2 smallish Granny Smith or other juicy, tart apples
⅓ cup Splenda
2 tablespoons Sucanat

Preheat the oven to 350°F. Spray an 8-inch-square baking dish with nonstick cooking spray.

Combine the dry ingredients in your food processor (with the S-blade in place) and pulse quickly to mix. Then add the butter, cut into a few chunks. Pulse till the butter is cut in.

Dump half of this mixture into your baking dish and press it into an even layer. Dump the rest of the grain mixture into a bowl for the time being. Put the food processor bowl back on the base, and put the S-blade back in.

Cut your apples into quarters and cut out the cores and stem. Throw the quarters into the food processor and pulse till they're chopped medium-fine.

Layer the apples over the grain mixture in the pan. Sprinkle the Splenda and Sucanat evenly over them. Then crumble the remaining grain mixture over the apples.

Bake for 35 minutes; then cool a bit before cutting.

9 servings, each with 260 calories, 15 g fat, 16 g protein, 17 g carbohydrate, 4 g fiber

Yummy Apple-Walnut Cake-Pie Thing

Is it a pie? Is it a cake? Who cares? It's irresistible.

> ¼ cup Sucanat
> ¾ cup Splenda
> ¼ cup almond meal
> ¼ cup vanilla whey protein powder
> 1 teaspoon baking powder
> ⅛ teaspoon salt
> 1 egg
> ½ teaspoon vanilla extract
> 2 medium apples, peeled, cored, and chopped
> ½ cup chopped walnuts

Preheat the oven to 350°F. Spray a 9-inch pie plate with non-stick cooking spray.

In a broad and shallow mixing bowl, combine the Sucanat, Splenda, almond meal, vanilla whey protein, baking powder, and salt. Stir together to distribute evenly.

Now beat the egg with the vanilla, then pour it into the dry ingredients. Stir till everything is evenly moist—mixture will be thick and sticky. Stir in the apples and walnuts.

Spread mixture in your prepared pie plate, and bake for 30 minutes.

8 servings, each with 161 calories, 7 g fat, 9 g protein, 17 g carbohydrate, 2 g fiber

Appendix A

Glycemic Loads of Common Foods

Food Item	Description	Available Carbohydrate (%)	Typical Serving	Glycemic Load
Lab standard:				
white bread	30 g	47	N/A	100
Baked Goods				
Oatmeal cookie	1 medium	68	1 oz.	102
Apple muffin, sugarless	2½-in. diameter	32	2½ oz.	107
Cookie: average, all types	1 medium	64	1 oz.	114
Croissant	1 medium	46	1½ oz.	127
Crumpet	1 medium	38	2 oz.	148
Bran muffin	2½-in. diameter	42	2 oz.	149
Pastry	Average serving	46	2 oz.	149
Chocolate cake	1 slice (4″ x 4″ x 1″)	47	3 oz.	154
Vanilla wafers	4 wafers	72	1 oz.	159
Graham cracker	1 rectangle	72	1 oz.	159
Blueberry muffin	2½-in. diameter	51	2 oz.	169
Pita	1 medium	57	2 oz.	189
Carrot cake	1 square (3″ x 3″ x 1½″)	56	2 oz.	199
Carrot muffin	2½-in. diameter	56	2 oz.	199

Food Item	Description	Available Carbohydrate (%)	Typical Serving	Glycemic Load
Baked Goods (continued)				
Waffle	7-in. diameter	37	2½ oz.	203
Doughnut	1 medium	49	2 oz.	205
Cupcake	2½-in. diameter	68	1½ oz.	213
Angel food cake	1 slice (4″ x 4″ x 1″)	58	2 oz.	216
English muffin	1 medium	47	2 oz.	224
Pound cake	1 slice (4″ x 4″ x 1″)	53	3 oz.	241
Corn muffin	2½-in. diameter	51	2 oz.	299
Pancake	5-in. diameter	73	2½ oz.	346
Alcoholic Beverages				
Spirits	1½ oz.	0	1½ oz.	<15
Red wine	6-oz. glass	0	6 oz.	<15
White wine	6-oz. glass	0	6 oz.	<15
Beer	12-oz. can/ bottle	3	12 oz.	<15
Nonalcoholic Beverages				
Tomato juice	8-oz. glass	4	8 oz.	36
Chocolate milk	8-oz. glass	10	8 oz.	82
Carrot juice	8-oz. glass	12	8 oz.	91
Grapefruit juice, unsweetened	8-oz. glass	9	8 oz.	100
Apple juice, unsweetened	8-oz. glass	12	8 oz.	109
Orange juice	8-oz. glass	10	8 oz.	119
Raspberry smoothie	8-oz. glass	16	8 oz.	127
Cranberry juice	8-oz. glass	12	8 oz.	145
Pineapple juice, unsweetened	8-oz. glass	14	8 oz.	145
Coca-Cola	12-oz. can	10	12 oz.	218
Gatorade	20-oz. bottle	6	20 oz.	273
Orange soda	12-oz. can	14	12 oz.	314

Breads and Rolls

Tortilla, wheat	1 medium	52	1¾ oz.	80
Pizza crust	1 slice	22	3½ oz.	70
White bread	1 slice, ½ in. thick	47	1 oz.	107
Wholemeal rye bread	⅜-in. slice	40	2 oz.	114
Sourdough bread	⅜-in. slice	47	1½ oz.	114
Tortilla, corn	1 medium	48	1¾ oz.	120
Oat bran bread	⅜-in. slice	60	1½ oz.	128
Whole wheat bread	1 slice, ½ in. thick	43	1½ oz.	129
Light rye bread	⅜-in. slice	47	1½ oz.	142
Banana bread, sugarless	1 slice (4″ x 4″ x 1″)	48	3 oz.	170
80% whole-kernel oat bread	⅜-in. slice	63	1½ oz.	170
Pita	8-in. diameter	57	2 oz.	189
Hamburger bun	Top and bottom, 5-in. diameter	50	2½ oz.	213
80% whole-kernel wheat bread	⅜-in. slice	67	2¼ oz.	213
French bread	1 slice, ½ in. thick	50	2 oz.	284
Bagel	1 medium	50	3⅓ oz.	340

Breakfast Cereals

All-Bran	½ cup	77	1 oz.	85
Muesli	1 cup	53	1 oz.	95
Special K	1 cup	70	1 oz.	133
Cheerios	1 cup	40	1 oz.	142
Shredded wheat	1 cup	67	1 oz.	142
Grape-Nuts	1 cup	70	1 oz.	142
Puffed wheat	1 cup	70	1 oz.	151
Instant oatmeal (cooked)	1 cup	10	8 oz.	154
Cream of Wheat (cooked)	1 cup	10	8 oz.	154
Total	1 cup	73	1 oz.	161

Food Item	Description	Available Carbohydrate (%)	Typical Serving	Glycemic Load
Breakfast Cereals (continued)				
Cornflakes	1 cup	77	1 oz.	199
Rice Krispies	1 cup	87	1 oz.	208
Rice Chex	1 cup	87	1 oz.	218
Raisin bran	1 cup	63	2 oz.	227
Candy				
Life Saver	1 piece	100	⅒ oz.	20
Peanut M&M's	1 snack-size package	57	¾ oz.	43
White chocolate	2 squares (1″ x 1″ x ¼″)	44	⅔ oz.	49
Chocolate	2 squares (1″ x 1″ x ¼″)	44	1 oz.	68
Snickers bar	1 regular-size bar	57	2 oz.	218
Jelly beans	⅓ cup	93	1½ oz.	312
Chips and Crackers				
Potato chips	1 small bag	42	1 oz.	62
Corn chips	1 package	52	1 oz.	97
Popcorn	4 cups	55	1 oz.	114
Rye crisps	1 rectangle	64	1 oz.	125
Wheat Thins	4 small	68	1 oz.	136
Soda cracker	2 regular-size	68	1 oz.	136
Pretzels	Small bag	67	1 oz.	151
Dairy Products				
Eggs	2 regular size	0	1½ oz.	<15
Cheese	1 slice (2″ x 2″ x 1″)	0	2 oz.	<15
Butter	1 tablespoon	0	¼ oz.	<15
Margarine	1 tablespoon	0	¼ oz.	<15
Sour cream	2 tablespoons	0	½ oz.	<15
Yogurt, plain unsweetened	½ cup	5	4 oz.	17

Milk, whole	8-oz. glass	5	8 oz.	27
Yogurt, low-fat sweetened	½ cup	16	4 oz.	57
Vanilla ice cream, high-fat	½ cup	18	4 oz.	68
Milk, low-fat chocolate	8-oz. glass	10	8 oz.	82
Vanilla ice cream, low-fat	½ cup	20	4 oz.	114
Frozen tofu dessert	½ cup	30	4 oz.	379

Fruit

Strawberries	1 cup	3	5½ oz.	13
Apricot	1 medium	8	2 oz.	24
Grapefruit	1 half	9	4½ oz.	32
Plum	1 medium	10	3 oz.	36
Kiwifruit	1 medium	10	3 oz.	43
Peach	1 medium	9	4 oz.	47
Grapes	1 cup (40 grapes)	15	2½ oz.	47
Pineapple	1 slice (¾″ thick x 3½″ diam.)	11	3 oz.	50
Watermelon	1 cup cubed	5	5½ oz.	52
Pear	1 medium	9	6 oz.	57
Mango	½ cup	14	3 oz.	57
Orange	1 medium	9	6 oz.	71
Apple	1 medium	13	5½ oz.	78
Banana	1 medium	17	3¼ oz.	85
Raisins	2 tablespoons	73	1 oz.	133
Figs	3 medium	43	2 oz.	151
Dates	5 medium	67	1½ oz.	298

Meat

Beef	10-oz. steak	0	10 oz.	<15
Pork	2 5-oz. chops	0	10 oz.	<15
Chicken	1 breast	0	10 oz.	<15
Fish	8-oz. fillet	0	8 oz.	<15
Lamb	3 4-oz. chops	0	12 oz.	<15

Food Item	Description	Available Carbohydrate (%)	Typical Serving	Glycemic Load
Nuts				
Peanuts	¼ cup	8	1¼ oz.	7
Cashews	¼ cup	26	1¼ oz.	21
Pasta				
Asian bean noodles	1 cup	25	5 oz.	118
Wholemeal spaghetti	1 cup	23	5 oz.	126
Vermicelli	1 cup	24	5 oz.	126
Spaghetti (boiled 5 min.)	1 cup	27	5 oz.	142
Fettucine	1 cup	23	5 oz.	142
Noodles, instant (cooked 2 min.)	1 cup	22	5 oz.	150
Capellini	1 cup	25	5 oz.	158
Spaghetti (boiled 10–15 min.)	1 cup	27	5 oz.	166
Couscous	½ cup	23	4 oz.	174
Linguine	1 cup	25	5 oz.	181
Macaroni	1 cup	28	5 oz.	181
Rice noodles	1 cup	22	5 oz.	181
Spaghetti (boiled 20 min.)	1 cup	24	5 oz.	213
Macaroni and cheese (boxed)	1 cup	28	5 oz.	252
Gnocchi	1 cup	27	5 oz.	260
Soups				
Tomato soup	1 cup	7	8 oz.	55
Minestrone	1 cup	7	8 oz.	64
Lentil soup	1 cup	8	8 oz.	82
Split pea soup	1 cup	11	8 oz.	145
Black bean soup	1 cup	11	8 oz.	154

Sweeteners

Artificial sweeteners	1 teaspoon	0	⅙ oz.	<15
Honey	1 teaspoon	72	⅙ oz.	16
Table sugar	1 round teaspoon	100	⅙ oz.	28
Syrup	¼ cup	100	2 oz.	364

Vegetables

Asparagus	4 spears	6	3 oz.	<15
Broccoli	½ cup	6	1½ oz.	<15
Cucumber	1 cup	2	6 oz.	<15
Lettuce	1 cup	3	2½ oz.	<15
Mushrooms	½ cup	7	2 oz.	<15
Bell pepper	½ medium	4	2 oz.	<15
Spinach	1 cup	5	2½ oz.	<15
Tornato	1 medium	6	5 oz.	<15
Peas	¼ cup	9	1½ oz.	16
Carrot (raw)	1 medium (7½-in. length)	10	3 oz.	21
Carrot (boiled)	½ cup	13	3½ oz.	33
Kidney beans	½ cup	17	3 oz.	40
Navy beans	½ cup	10	3 oz.	40
Garbanzo beans	½ cup	20	3 oz.	45
Lima beans	½ cup	12	3 oz.	57
Pinto beans	½ cup	17	3 oz.	57
Black-eyed peas	½ cup	20	3 oz.	74
Yam	½ cup	24	5 oz.	123
Potato (instant mashed)	¾ cup	13	5 oz.	161
Baked potato	1 medium	20	5 oz.	246
Sweet potato	½ cup	19	5 oz.	161
Corn on the cob	1 ear	21	5⅓ oz.	171
French fries	Medium serving (McDonald's)	19	5¼ oz.	219
Baked potato	1 medium	20	5 oz.	246

Food Item	Description	Available Carbohydrate (%)	Typical Serving	Glycemic Load
Rice				
Rice cakes	1 medium size	84	1 oz.	193
Brown rice	1 cup	22	6½ oz.	222
Basmati rice	1 cup	25	6½ oz.	271
White rice	1 cup	24	6½ oz.	283
Miscellaneous				
Salad dressing	2 tablespoons	6	1 oz.	<15

Appendix B

Converting to Metrics

Volume Measurement Conversions

U.S.	Metric
¼ teaspoon	1.25 ml
½ teaspoon	2.5 ml
¾ teaspoon	3.75 ml
1 teaspoon	5 ml
1 tablespoon	15 ml
¼ cup	62.5 ml
½ cup	125 ml
¾ cup	187.5 ml
1 cup	250 ml

Weight Measurement Conversions

U.S.	Metric
1 ounce	28.4 g
8 ounces	227.5 g
16 ounces (1 pound)	455 g

Cooking Temperature Conversions

Celsius/Centigrade: 0°C and 100°C are placed arbitrarily at the melting and boiling points of water and standard to the metric system.

Fahrenheit: Fahrenheit established 0°F as the stabilized temperature when equal amounts of ice, water, and salt are mixed.

To convert temperatures in Fahrenheit to Celsius, use this formula:

$$C = (F - 32) \times 0.5555$$

So, for example, if you are baking at 350°F and want to know that temperature in Celsius, use this calculation:

$$C = (350 - 32) \times 0.5555 = 176.65°C$$

Index

About the Authors

Dr. Rob Thompson is a graduate of the University of Washington School of Medicine. He completed a residency in internal medicine and a fellowship in cardiology at the University of Illinois at Chicago and served as director of the coronary care unit at Harborview Hospital in Seattle before entering private practice in 1977. For the past twenty-five years, he has specialized in preventive cardiology, the treatment of conditions that lead to blood-vessel disease, including high blood cholesterol, obesity, and diabetes. He is the author of *The New Low-Carb Way of Life* (New York: M. Evans, 2002) and *The Glycemic-Load Diet* (Chicago: McGraw-Hill, 2006). He has published several articles in medical journals, including original contributions in *The Journal of the American Medical Association* and *The Annals of Internal Medicine*. Since medical school, Dr. Thompson has had an abiding interest in uncovering and correcting the underlying causes of diseases. He considers obesity and diabetes "diseases of civilization," caused and worsened by conditions characteristic of the modern lifestyle that, he believes, do not require unusual willpower to correct.

Dr. Thompson lives with his wife in Seattle. They are parents of two grown children. He is an avid skier, golfer, and fly fisher.

Additional information about the glycemic-load diet can be found at Dr. Thompson's website, lowglycemicload.com.

Dana Carpender, author of eight cookbooks, including the best-selling *500 Low-Carb Recipes*, started her writing career as a self-published author. In 1995, after years of creative low-fat cooking featuring whole grains and other "healthy" carbohydrates, and despite five-step aerobics classes per week, she found herself a size 20, and gaining! Worse, her blood pressure was rising, and she was left dragging by energy swings. Dropping carbs long before it was fashionable, Carpender lost forty pounds with no hunger, achieved normal blood pressure and excellent blood lipids, and found herself with more energy in her forties than she'd had in her teens.

Taking her long-time fascination with nutrition and a passion for sharing that life-changing experience of going low carb, Carpender wrote *How I Gave Up My Low-Fat Diet and Lost 40 Pounds* and started started *Lowcarbezine!* a weekly online newsletter, to help spread the word. That self-published book netted Carpender a publishing deal that led to the bestselling *500 Low-Carb Recipes* and all the books that have followed.

All of this has established Carpender as the knowledgeable, funny, and occasionally opinionated Everywoman who knows how to make eating healthy fun, easy, and delicious. *500 Low-Carb Recipes*, published by Fair Winds Press in 2002, has sold more than 500,000 copies to date and won the Carbohydrate Awareness Council's Consumer's Choice Award for best cookbook of 2003. Her other books include *15 Minute Low-Carb Recipes*, *500 More Low-Carb Recipes*, *The Low-Carb Barbecue Book*, *Low-Carb Smoothies*, a revised, expanded edition of *How I Gave Up My Low-Fat Diet and Lost 40 Pounds*, and her latest, the *Every Calorie Counts Cookbook*, featuring recipes that take both calorie count and glycemic impact into account. In January 2008, Carpender traded *Lowcarbezine!* for a blog at www.holdthetoast .com, where she writes about all aspects of low-carb living, and especially about low-carb cooking.

Carpender appears frequently on television, radio, and in print across the country. Her appearances have included *Weekend Today*, *Fox and Friends*, *The Wayne Brady Show*, and many appearances on QVC. Print credits include *Woman's Day*, *Low Carb Energy*, and the *National Enquirer*.

Never embracing the "meat and eggs only" philosophy, Carpender's recipes feature a bountiful harvest of fruits and vegetables; every variety of protein, nuts and seeds; healthy fats and a wide variety of flavors from around the world. Knowing that bodies have differing tolerances, she offers alternatives whenever possible, letting readers adjust the carbohydrate and calorie levels to their own needs. Her instructions are clear and concise, and occasionally funny.

A fierce proponent of real, nutritious foods, Carpender also emphasizes that regardless of carbohydrate or calorie count, everything we eat should serve our health. She examines the nutritional value of all types of foods, while taking into account people's needs for practical meal solutions and short-cut preparations.

Carpender lives in Bloomington, Indiana, with her husband and four pets, all of whom eschew junk food. When she's not cooking, writing, or reading the latest nutrition research, she power-walks, reads mystery novels, and is an enthusiastic Toastmaster, taking the occasional trophy. You can write to her at dana@hold thetoast.com.